Unmasked

Unmasked

COVID, Community, and
the Case of Okoboji

Emily Mendenhall

VANDERBILT UNIVERSITY PRESS
Nashville, Tennessee

Portions of this work were originally published in a slightly different form as "How an Iowa Summer Resort Region Became a Covid-19 Hot Spot," Vox.com, August 8, 20120, www.vox.com/2020/8/8/21357625/covid-19-iowa-lakes-okoboji-kim-reynolds-masks. Used by permission of Vox Media, LLC.

Library of Congress Cataloging-in-Publication Data

Names: Mendenhall, Emily, 1982– author.
Title: Unmasked : covid, community, and the case of Okoboji / Emily Mendenhall.
Description: Nashville, Tennessee : Vanderbilt University Press, 2022. | Includes bibliographical references and index.
Identifiers: LCCN 2021040748 (print) | LCCN 2021040749 (ebook) | ISBN 9780826504524 (hardcover) | ISBN 9780826504531 (epub) | ISBN 9780826504548 (pdf)
Subjects: LCSH: COVID-19 Pandemic, 2020– | COVID-19 (Disease) | Okoboji (Iowa)
Classification: LCC RA644.C67 M463 2022 (print) | LCC RA644.C67 (ebook) | DDC 362.1962/414009777123—dc23/eng/20211015

LC record available at https://lccn.loc.gov/2021040748
LC ebook record available at https://lccn.loc.gov/2021040749

For Bubs, for Mamoo
For our family

CONTENTS

A NOTE ON NAMES

ALL NAMES AND identifying details have been changed to protect the confidentiality of those I interviewed formally for this research. I use pseudonyms and indicate so in the text, which is common practice among anthropologists. I have not anonymized my family members. I also have not changed the names of public figures, including business owners and elected officials. In many cases, I cite their public writing, interviews, and comments on the events throughout the summer recorded elsewhere; this is especially true among those individuals who declined to speak with me. However, I have changed the names of school board members whose views I recorded in public forums. I quoted some of these community leaders in an article I wrote for *Vox* in August 2020, just before they voted on masking for the school year—a period of intense community tension. I hope providing some anonymity for these leaders here impedes bringing those feelings back to the surface.

PROLOGUE

WRITING ABOUT YOUR hometown can be tricky. Especially when some of what you write may be unflattering.
For five generations my family has resided in northwest
Iowa, along the shores of West Lake Okoboji in the Iowa
Great Lakes region.[1] My great-grandparents bought some
lakefront property from a businessman trying to make a
quick buck in 1907. Over several decades they built a summer retreat with little cabins hugging the lakeshore. They
bought another lot and eventually built a small family
resort to which my grandparents devoted their lives, selling it only two years before my older sister was born. My
father grew up on the shores of West Lake Okoboji and
eventually instilled in me a similar love of the peaceful
waters that run through his veins. I lived there too, until
I left to study at a small college on the east coast.

This book is about balancing perspective. Although
now I've lived far from Okoboji as long as I lived there, the
community is part of who I am. I have evangelized for these
waters all over the world, dropping "OKOBOJI" towels,
cups, and t-shirts for mentors, friends, and colleagues. Yet,

as my ideas about the world grew bigger, and my experiences deeper, how I conceive a community that gave me so much has changed enormously.

When I left home to attend Davidson College, my unfamiliarity with the way things worked made me realize how little I knew about the world. I had to relearn American and world history because what I had learned growing up had been a heavily edited version. I read people's stories and histories from the perspectives of those who lived them in courses in literature, anthropology, sociology, and philosophy. I also spent months in mentored courses in Nicaragua, Chile, and Zambia, which opened my eyes to the different ways people live in the world, and trained me to truly listen and learn from others in a deeper way than I had ever done before. I realized that people live in very different cultural contexts, even in the United States; many of my classmates came from private schools or wealthy Southern families that were very different from mine. I'm a happy-go-lucky type of person, so I jumped in with both feet. But there were some aspects of Davidson College that made me uneasy (such as blatant differences in how students experienced the college based on race, class, gender, and sexuality). Despite my seeing and experiencing some of these things (re: sexism), as a cisgender white female I also realized how much advantage came with the parts of my person that I could not control (as others also could not).

I am now a medical anthropologist and professor at Georgetown University in Washington, DC, where I often tell my students that your twenties are for becoming who you are (listening, learning) and your thirties are for creating (making, sharing). In my twenties I completed two graduate degrees: one in public health and another in anthropology. I spent five years in Chicago, working at Cook County Hospital, learning about how trauma can become embodied in chronic illness from Mexican immigrant women seeking care there.[2] I also spent years living outside the United States, accruing treasured mentors and experiences in India, Kenya, South Africa, and the United Kingdom; these mentors, along with the meaningful work I've been privileged to do, have shaped who I am and how I see the world.[3] I bring together these perspectives in my research, in understanding what people struggle with and where (public health) and why and how people struggle with illness differently in one place as opposed to another (anthropology). I have interviewed hundreds of people (mostly women) around the world, trying to understand what makes people sick and why.

Yet, I have never missed an Okoboji summer. Even when my visits were brief, going home was comforting in part because I grew up next door to my British grandmother (my mother's mother), who showered me with love in her austere and proper way. After her husband died when she was in her early fifties, she returned many times to London to visit her family, while also traveling around the world during the bitterly cold prairie winters in Iowa. She inspired in me a passion for understanding places far away from my home, even when many people around me remained somewhat insular. We stayed very close until she died, just six weeks after my youngest daughter was born. Since she passed away, I have had a difficult time connecting with my home.

But when coronavirus spread throughout the world, and my family became integral to the COVID-19 response in Dickinson County in the Iowa Great Lakes region, my personal and professional life came together. This crisis drew me back to the community.

This book is the story of what happened during one Okoboji summer when a pandemic reached northwest Iowa, forcing the community to face a global challenge. My research and writing about this challenge cannot be divorced from my professional and personal identities. I work and live in a global community of scholars and policymakers who are constantly discussing how people, viruses, histories, and politics are interconnected. I continue to dedicate my professional life to understanding these challenges.

Yet I come from a place that can be frustratingly insular and isolationist, even though it certainly is not an island, bubble, or escape from reality. My family lives there and is deeply embedded in this community—giving hours of their time to community service, investing in the future of the community's children, and carefully monitoring the waters to ensure future generations can safely live in and on the sacred shores. I recognize and honor the advantages the community has given me—the wealth my family gained by purchasing land before tourism drove up property values, growing up in a tight-knit community where

I knew people cared for me, and having a public school system that enabled me to achieve my goals.

But there is still a need to understand and critique the devaluation of life that emerged during the summer when people faced an extraordinary question in the face of a virus: How do we care for each other?

CHAPTER 1

GLOBAL THREATS

I FIRST REALIZED that coronavirus might upend our lives one Tuesday afternoon when Dr. Rebecca Katz stopped by my office. It was March 3, 2020, and she was bustling through the Intercultural Center at Georgetown University. As she swept by, she popped her head into my office as she usually does to say hi.

We are professors who work on very different questions in global health at the Walsh School of Foreign Service (SFS) at Georgetown University. I am a medical anthropologist who studies how people perceive and experience illness, particularly when it is new or foreign to them. Rebecca is an expert in global health security. When coronavirus became a real threat, her phone never stopped ringing. She was the first to raise her eyebrows to me about the news from Wuhan, China, where coronavirus began to spread in December of 2019. Back in January of 2020, she started talking with our colleague and global health law expert Alexandra Phelan about the whispers.[1] They became concerned. I grilled her about what she knew, from where, and what was our risk for it coming to the US.

"I've cancelled my travel for the next three months," Rebecca said as she texted something on her phone. "Beth Cameron came back from a conference last week super sick. I'm not taking any chances." She had one foot in my office and the other in the hall. She sighed as she leaned against my door in her smart leather jacket. Beth Cameron was not only a good friend of Rebecca's but also the lead of the Global Health Security Agenda for the Obama administration—clearly, they were talking about this outbreak becoming serious.

"Wait, really?" I responded.

"Yeah, hold on a minute. I have to get back to the president."

In 2014, during my first year working at SFS, I realized I was entering a whole new world when Angela Stent, a professor of East European studies and expert on Russia, rushed late into a faculty meeting. She apologized; she had been speaking with the president. I nearly spat my lemonade across the table. She was advising the White House after Russia invaded Crimea, a part of Ukraine. I quickly realized how frequently my colleagues consult on issues of national and international security, providing regional and technical expertise.

But Rebecca had been speaking with Jack DeGioia, Georgetown's president. She was one of five experts gathered to discuss a number of key questions that would inform the next steps for the university in the face of an uncertain pandemic. Already DeGioia was bringing together experts to figure out what to do. What is the risk on campus? How many new cases are in DC (incidence)? How many cases were recorded in the past week (prevalence)? Where are they clustering? Should we close down campus? Do we stay open? Do we pack up students and send them home? All students, or some? What if it's not safe for them to go home? What if students don't have space to think, grow, and study? How do we close down or stay partially open and make things equitable? Where do they stay?

Spring break began in three days. Students were planning to trek across the United States and the globe for academic programs and personal travel. We weren't sure what to do.

The university closed down a week later. We taught virtually for the next year.

SECURITIZE

Before I describe what happened in my hometown, I am going to tell you Rebecca's story. Her life shows how Americans had for decades planned for a viral threat like SARS-CoV-2—also known as the novel coronavirus or coronavirus disease (COVID-19)—which could shut down airports, shutter businesses, send kids home from school, and devastate families. I heard her describe more times than I can remember how a global pandemic could not only devastate the economy but also upend people's lives in irreversible ways. For years she worked feverishly developing pandemic preparedness plans in part with the Obama administration. But these plans were forgotten soon after President Trump took office.

Over a double espresso one afternoon, Rebecca told me she had been thinking about infectious disease since she was in third grade. She grew up in a house where her parents were completely entwined in the science of HIV and AIDS. Her father, Fred Katz, a hematologist and blood banker, spent his career at the American Red Cross. Fred Katz was on TV so much during her childhood that he had his own video camera at home. This was unusual because it was the 1980s, when few people had computers let alone video cameras. But these were unusual times. The HIV crisis caused extraordinary stress and uncertainty around the world, and Americans who lived through that time cannot forget the fear many people had about what the virus was and who was infected or infectious. HIV was so stigmatizing that some people suggested marking those who tested positive by tattooing them on the face. But Fred Katz was as calm talking about blood supply during the AIDS pandemic as he was talking about the weather. Fred's contributions were well documented in a full spread in *People* magazine in 1983 and the iconic movie of the early years of the AIDS epidemic that came out a decade later, *And the Band Played On.*

Rebecca's mother was anything but calm and quiet. Deborah Katz started her career at the National Institutes of Health (NIH) AIDS division in 1982, where she worked with Dr. Anthony Fauci, the director of the National Institute of Allergy and Infectious Diseases. She stayed for thirty years. Early on in her career, she managed the politics of a clinical trial amid the AIDS crisis in America—navigating who could be enrolled, when, and for how long. At the time, many people from the gay community were dying from Kaposi sarcoma, a rare cancer that develops when people's conditions advance to AIDS (acquired immunodeficiency syndrome). In fact, so many gay men were infected with the new virus that scientists initially called HIV (the virus), GRID—gay-related immune deficiency, a stigmatizing term associating the virus with homosexuality.[2] Debbie was often called in the middle of the night to finagle people into studies, particularly those who got really sick fast. It was a time of extraordinary fear and uncertainty.

The 1980s were all-engrossing for scientists studying HIV and AIDS. With both parents working nonstop on HIV, dinner conversations in the Katz household concerned what was going on with research, people, and treatment. Rebecca once said to me, while walking on the C&O Trail along the Potomac River, "my sister and I grew up knowing more about HIV in the eighties than any kid who didn't have it." But many people were not as empathetic or understanding and instead feared the new illness. She recalled a plumber entering their house and seeing a huge poster on the fridge that said, "Women don't get AIDS, they die of AIDS." He turned around and left. Observing this kind of fear shaped Rebecca's childhood and cultivated an awareness of what viral threats can do.

In the *People* spread, Fred Katz said, "AIDS hysteria is potentially as lethal as the disease itself."[3] In both the AIDS and COVID-19 pandemics, the early days introduced a great deal of fear and disbelief because people knew so little about who was getting sick, from where, and why.[4] Naming and blaming were as common in the early days of the HIV pandemic as they were within the early days of the COVID-19 pandemic.[5] Not unlike the early stigmatization of the gay community in the early days of HIV, the Sinophobia experienced by many Asian Americans was intensified throughout the COVID-19 pandemic. This xenophobia stemmed in part from President Trump's unremitting use of "China virus" and "Wuhan virus" in lieu of coronavirus or COVID-19 to politically spar with another superpower and blame it for the pandemic.[6] The consequences of this political gamesmanship were extraordinary for many Americans who faced unrelenting racism throughout the pandemic period.

There were also many political similarities between HIV and SARS-CoV-2, and I will only mention a few here. For years the Reagan administration ignored the severity of HIV, joking at times about who was dying and why. It wasn't until the virus spread throughout the country and deaths surged that many scientists and political officials took HIV and AIDS seriously.[7] Similarly, the Trump administration ignored the severity of coronavirus in the United States for most of 2020, suggesting it was "just the flu" and would "go away."[8] In both cases, political negligence could not stymie pioneering medical innovation, which was fueled by unprecedented political activism, money, and urgency. Anti-retroviral therapy (ART) that prolonged life for people living with HIV was developed in five years, changing what was formerly a death sentence into a survivable chronic illness in America.[9] Coronavirus would see a vaccine within one year—a timeline unfathomable to scientists and the public alike only months before.[10] But who reaped the benefits of these technologies and when was similarly uneven: profits were prioritized over people's lives and pharmaceutical companies were reluctant to waive patents, thereby making it difficult to make more medicines at lower costs that could reach people around the world.[11] These challenges for global health equity remain enormous and reveal why Rebecca's work matters so much.[12]

Growing up in the time of AIDS had a huge impact on Rebecca. But so did her own infection. Rebecca caught *Brucella melitensis* while working in a maternal and child health clinic in Karnataka, a state in southern India. It took months to figure out what had made her sick and years to recover. She discovered her infection had been the first agent ever weaponized by the US bioweapons program in 1950. She became obsessed with studying what her disease was, how it was used, and the role diseases played in international politics. This led Rebecca to work on biosecurity at the State Department for fifteen years, asking hard questions: Why do some diseases cause a global stir and others don't? How do diseases travel across the globe so quickly? What do nations need to do to prepare for the next viral intruder?

I tell her story because Rebecca is one of a handful of academics and practitioners who came together to fuel a movement to put global health security on the national agenda. Rebecca strategized with others in a series of meetings in the Eisenhower Executive Office Buildings next to the White House in 2013. They discussed "what comes next" after President Barack Obama gave two speeches that mentioned global health security.

In 2009, President Obama encouraged countries to work together on many efforts, including health, women's rights, science, and security, in what is known as the Cairo Speech. The global health security community, including Rebecca, was thrilled by the recognition of how a viral threat could bring the country to a halt. President Obama stated, "Governments that protect these rights are ultimately more stable, successful and secure. Suppressing ideas never succeeds in making them go away."[13]

Two years later, when addressing the United Nations General Assembly, President Obama spoke of countries coming together and the significance of the International Health Regulations, or IHR. The IHR is an international law that coordinates disease surveillance and global cooperation in the response to outbreaks. The law is decades old, but has been rewritten with increasing concern as viral threats intensified: Ebola. SARS. Avian flu. Lassa fever. Chikungunya.[14]

The IHR outlines the rules for trade and travel, as well as hygiene and surveillance, when new viruses spread across borders. In many ways, legal solutions through IHR have become a fixture in facing many risks—from humans, animals, and ecosystems—that contribute to viral threats.[15] Rebecca wrote with our Georgetown colleague Lawrence Gostin in the *Milbank Quarterly* that the IHR is critical for responding to rapid shifts in the modern world that are now framed as "security risks" for countries who previously had few exposures to such viral threats.[16] The regulations demonstrate how emerging infections are inherently political problems.

By 2012, only 22 percent of countries had implemented the IHR. The Obama administration launched the Global

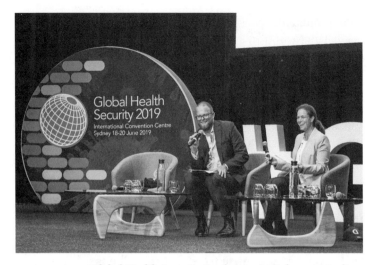

FIGURE 1.1. Global Health Security Conference in Sydney, Australia, 2019. Photography by Camera Creations, Sydney, Australia.

Health Security Agenda (GHSA) in February of 2014 to raise health security on the political agenda. The GHSA caused heads of states to talk about and marshal resources to address global health security. But by then, Rebecca had moved to Georgetown University, where we eventually met. She began to pull away from GHSA because it had become something it was not intended to be. It was meant to break down silos by bringing together funding, policy, and people to fight viral threats together. Instead, it created its own with action packages that siloed funding exclusively to the program. It was designed to strengthen the IHR, but in the end, it competed with it. It took on a life of its own.

This is a common story in global health, where priority agendas get more money and political attention. Where technological solutions, like vaccines, are prioritized over social ones, like masking, hand washing, and quarantining.[17] Where politics take priority over science.

President Trump dissolved the office in 2018.[18] Two years later, the country would be sideswiped by a virus for which Rebecca and others had written a pandemic playbook. Despite all this expertise and careful planning, their work was largely ignored.

HOW DID WE GET HERE?

Experts like Rebecca were not surprised by the novel coronavirus's emergence. They had warned the global community amid other regional outbreaks, such as SARS, Severe Acute Respiratory Syndrome. Michael Lemonick and Alice Park wrote in *Time* magazine in 2003, "If Americans think that they have dodged the biological bullet, they had better think again. As the truth about SARS comes out—slowly, due in large part to government cover-ups in the land of its birth—it is becoming clear that what is taking place in Asia threatens the entire world. Epidemiologists have long worried about a highly contagious, fatal disease that could spread quickly around the globe, and SARS might end up confirming their worst fears. Microbes can go wherever jet airliners do these days, so it is a very real possibility that the disease has not yet shown its full fury."[19]

America is the home of some of the best scientists in the world. Yet many of the international scientists who gave the United States the highest possible ranking for pandemic preparedness in a 2019 report underplayed how politics can trump science.[20] By February 2, 2020, Trump said, "We pretty much shut it down coming from China." By late February, he pontificated, "The Coronavirus is very much under control in the USA. . . . Stock Market [is] starting to look very good to me!" He repeated that it would "go away" or "disappear," often stating "this is a flu." By March 10, Trump continued, "Just stay calm. It will go away."[21] The next day the World Health Organization officially made the assessment that the coronavirus could be characterized as a pandemic.[22]

We knew science was being sidelined in the spring when Dr. Fauci, who served seven presidents, planted his face in his palm on national television. Why would Trump ignore or even try to smear someone who had helped America tackle the AIDS epidemic for decades? Journalists Peter Nicholas and Ed Yong wrote in the *Atlantic*,

> Targeting Fauci seems like a tragic misuse of White House time and energy if officials' aim is to defeat the coronavirus. But Trump appears more concerned with discrediting Fauci. [. . .] As much as Trump wants and needs Americans to see the virus as a nuisance that's soon to be overcome, Fauci is a recurring reminder that the crisis remains a grave and enduring threat, and that Trump has mishandled the pandemic. The Americans who believe the White House's anti-science campaign risk cutting themselves off from potentially life-saving information.[23]

Fauci quickly became a household name, but he wasn't in charge.

It soon became apparent that there would be no national strategy. Trump relegated power to the states, which created confusion, fear, and stress among many people across red and blue states alike. It was shocking to see a president who loved power so much pass the torch on the most consequential crisis of his presidency.[24] Yet, in many ways, giving states power to respond to the pandemic on their own terms illustrated his disillusion with government overreach (a central tenet of American conservatism). Putting power into the hands of governors also enabled the president to reward red states for supporting his messaging while condemning blue states by withholding funding or publicly admonishing them. For example, Trump threatened Democratic governors who condemned his handling of the pandemic, and coerced others into issuing public praise for his handling of the pandemic so he could use it in campaign ads.[25] Drew Altman argued in the *BMJ* that "delegating primary responsibility to the states in a crisis" resulted in "the states and the American peoples split strikingly along partisan lines in their response to COVID-19, as if the country has both red and blue pandemics."[26]

Iowa's governor, Kim Reynolds, was not threatened by Trump. Rather, she was embraced by him and governed in his image. This was not only because of conservative politics. Some people I spoke to thought "Corona Kim" was hoping to be the vice presidential candidate for Trump's reelection. Regardless of the motivations, local residents I spoke with believed Governor Reynolds did nothing. Although some did not think she could or should enforce Iowans to take COVID-19 risk seriously from the state level.

Iowa exemplifies what happens when leadership emphasizes personal responsibility during a crisis as opposed to

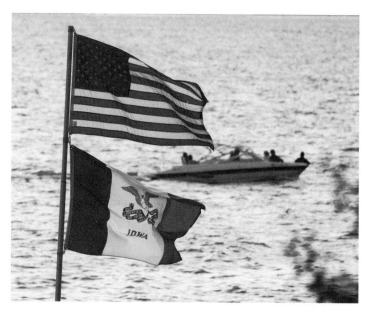

FIGURE 1.2. Iowa's flag. Courtesy of David Thoreson.

implementing policy.[27] Such rugged individualism is not
surprising; it's even inscribed on Iowa's state flag: "Our liberties we prize, and our rights we will maintain." But it's as
cultural as it is political. Economists have called the strong
antigovernment sentiments in the American Midwest a
"total frontier experience" that reveals a "primacy of personal goals over group goals and the regulation of behavior
by personal attitudes rather than social norms."[28] Midwestern historian Kristin Hoganson describes agrarian mar-
kets as bound into an "us-versus-them mentality, a desire
to dominate in a win-or-lose world."[29] Statements like "I
don't need the government," "I don't want the government
to interfere in my life," and "I don't trust the government"

are ubiquitous in the Iowa Great Lakes region and explain in part Reynolds's actions.

When Reynolds, like Trump, seemingly failed to set policy to guide how people should behave amid the greatest viral threat in a century, divergent social realities set in through which Iowans perceived risk and responsibility.[30] Some perceived coronavirus to be a death sentence: they knew someone who had died or who was at high risk for severe COVID-19 because of diabetes, hypertension, or a respiratory disease. Many used their health or youth as an excuse to live their lives uninhibited by the pandemic. Others prescribed to fatalism, thinking their future was predetermined, often by God. And some rejected the notion that the global viral threat was real at all.

CHAPTER 2

LOCATING OKOBOJI

ON MARCH 3, 2020, Lakes Regional Healthcare of Dickinson County, Iowa, posted the following message to their Facebook page:

> You've heard about it everywhere: coronavirus or COVID-19. Here Dr. Zach Borus tells you how to best prevent yourself from getting it, what to do to prepare for the possibility of getting it, how the hospital and clinic will care for you if you get it, and what sources to listen to. It's important to be alert but not anxious. Lakes Regional Healthcare and the clinics are well-prepared to care for any patients who may present with suspected or confirmed COVID-19.[1]

Linked to the message was Zach's first YouTube video about COVID-19 in the Iowa Great Lakes.[2] He introduced himself as a local physician at Lakes Regional Healthcare as well as president and medical director of the Dickinson County Board of Health. He described what the hospital was doing to prepare and introduced the virus to the community. He was calm and collected, and his thick beard, relaxed demeanor, and folksy language kept people at ease. Dr. Borus reminded the community to learn about the local coronavirus situation from health personnel as opposed to "willy-nilly on Facebook." The video was eight minutes and thirty-three seconds long.

Dr. Zachary Borus is also my brother-in-law. Zach and I started talking at length about coronavirus early on because we were concerned about our families. How do we protect our parents? Zach and my sister Kate live next door to my parents so we had constant conversations about their safety, especially in the early days when we knew so little about the virus. But my parents did not need so much advice. My dad had a busy urology practice in the community for more than thirty years. By 2020, both my parents were retired, although my father served on the Okoboji City Council and my mom served as treasurer for multiple community organizations. They did this from home. Most people in the community at that time embraced the mantra "we are all in this together" and did their part to keep neighbors safe from infection.

Zach is a family physician with a master's degree in public health, the two-year degree that trains you in epidemiology, prevention, and thinking about risk in communities (not just individuals). This focus on the community is a distinction from medicine; in medicine you are trained very narrowly to study one area of the body, one specific organ, one individual. For example, when I asked my obstetrician about severe sciatic pain after my second baby was born, she said, "I don't deal with the spine!" That's true among most physicians, as they specialize and think quite narrowly, focusing on diagnosing what's wrong in a system in a body. In contrast, public health focuses on the health of the community, recognizing that where people live, how they think, and what they do affects health.

Zach was attracted to family medicine precisely because it did not take a narrow approach to health. I cannot count the times over the years that I have called him to talk about a physical pain, my kids' scrapes, or my research. For the past sixteen years, I have studied how trauma and social distress over many years can contribute to depression and type 2 diabetes. I am also curious about how mental and physical health compound one another. This compounding effect means that if your body aches, then that ache affects your mind, and vice versa. Family medicine, especially in northwest Iowa, where the majority of sick patients are aging, deals with diabetes and other conditions of the heart, blood, kidneys, and brain. These are the chronic conditions that have surged in the past seventy years around the world and kill more people annually on a global scale than infections like HIV.[3]

Zach began convening with the medical community in February to discuss COVID-19. But few people projected the amount of virus that would come to the Iowa Great Lakes. By March, the medical and public health teams began meeting daily with the emergency management services for the county. They conducted the first COVID-19 test on March 10, 2020, although at that time only people with symptoms AND a comorbidity AND potential travel-related exposure were permitted to get tested. Their first case was found on March 16, 2020. This was the same day

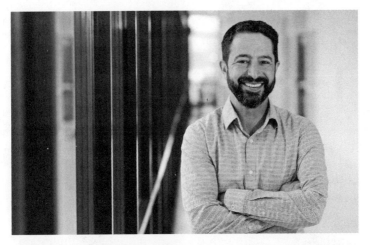

FIGURE 2.1. Zach Borus. Photo courtesy of *OKOBOJI* magazine.

schools shut down in the Iowa Great Lakes region for the remainder of the academic year.

The first case in Okoboji occurred at the same time as the big outbreaks in New York and Seattle. Hospitals in those cities were overrun with patients dying from COVID-19, and people on the coasts were panicked. Rebecca was constantly on the national news in an attempt to abate misinformation and fear.[4] I was in lockdown near DC, and my kids had a two-week break from school before virtual classes began. Schools went dark around the country and scrambled to serve up a virtual option as soon as they could. Families in the Iowa Great Lakes region were "all in this together" and stayed home for the next month, fearing an impending outbreak.

There was not a big outbreak that month in Okoboji, but there was in Worthington, Minnesota. Worthington is a forty-minute drive north and west from the Iowa Great

Lakes. Thirty people in Worthington tested positive by April 16 and at least seven had ties to the JBS Foods pork processing plant, which is central to the regional economy; they process twenty thousand pigs a day from Minnesota hog farmers.[5] That outbreak was on the heels of the major COVID-19 outbreak at the Smithfield Foods pork processing plant in Sioux Falls, South Dakota, which is another sixty miles west from Worthington. The Smithfield Foods outbreak caused hundreds of COVID-19 cases and at least one death by the time the JBS Foods plant had its first outbreak. The forty-two-year-old mayor of Sioux Falls, Paul TenHaken, said, "This thing jumped out of a light socket." It took a great deal of effort to make a giant pork producer shutter its doors, but the Republican mayor was even able to get the foot-dragging South Dakota governor to endorse the plant's shutdown. A week after the outbreak, 10 percent of Smithfield Foods employees tested positive, representing 40 percent of the coronavirus cases in South Dakota at the time.[6] This caused a great deal of panic in Okoboji because people move seamlessly between the Iowa Great Lakes region, Worthington, and Sioux Falls, which has the only Costco for miles. Yet with limited testing in Dickinson County and no large meat-packing operations, there was little worry that a huge outbreak would happen in the Iowa Great Lakes, as long as people continued to stay home.

THE LOCAL RESPONSE

The local stakes in preventing a coronavirus outbreak in the Iowa Great Lakes included both private and public players and state and local cooperation. The emergency management team, located at the courthouse on Hill Avenue in Spirit Lake, was a central player in coordinating the local response. The emergency management team usually deals with fires, drownings, and traffic concerns. COVID-19 posed an unusual challenge and required constant collaboration with health officials they had rarely worked with before. Emergency management worked closely with Lakes Regional Healthcare, where Zach worked, just down the road from the Courthouse. Lakes Regional Healthcare is the only hospital for thirty miles and is partly run by Dickinson County. Dickinson County Public Health is part of the hospital and serves the county, but it also responds to the Iowa Department of Public Health. Avera Medical Group, a private Catholic nonprofit headquartered in Sioux Falls, also has a stake in local healthcare. Avera partners with the local hospital to run the local family medicine clinic. These arrangements show how there are state, county, and private interests at play in public health management. It also indicates how our public health system is somewhat fragmented, with private and public stakes in what medicine is and how care functions. Each of these layers played a role in the coronavirus response in Dickinson County.

I reached out to Matt, who works in emergency management, after conducting several interviews, because everyone asked me, "Have you spoken to Matt?" We spoke in late July, more than a month after I had begun to poke my nose into the complexity of how people were thinking about the virus in Okoboji. I arrived a week after Memorial

Day amidst the first major spike in COVID-19 cases and dove into what anthropologists call "deep hanging out."[7] This means that I was embedded within the community in such a deep way that I was able to fold back the socio-cultural complexity behind what people thought, how they behaved, and why. I started texting my friends, sending notes on Facebook Messenger to classmates, and asking everyone I had known since childhood about what they thought about COVID and why. I wanted to understand why so few people were following public health recommendations in Okoboji.

As an anthropologist who studies the social experiences of epidemics, I could not help myself from delving deeper into the social phenomenon that was unfolding in front of me in my hometown. I interviewed eighty-six people formally for this research over the summer months and conducted several follow-up interviews with multiple study participants throughout the first pandemic year.[8] I observed public forums, exchanges, and behavior, often writing observations in my notebook, on my phone, or even on paper napkins when my kids had confiscated my cell. Throughout the book, I have anonymized quotes from people like Matt who I interviewed formally. I emailed Matt and we set up a time to talk.

Matt and I spoke over Zoom: he sat in his office at the courthouse and I was hidden away in my parents' basement, near a window. Matt explained how involved he had been in the coronavirus response for the county, though he had limited public health experience in the past. Matt explained, "I'm more on the response level so I try to keep politics out of this office as much as I can. It doesn't always happen. But, in general, [my job is] to put out house fires. Or I would go out to traffic accidents and help the traffic." Working on coronavirus was a new challenge, and different from traffic or a drowning. Everyone from locally elected officials to health providers said Matt was doing a good job with the coronavirus crisis: "talk to Matt!"

Matt was a notetaker and described his detailed daily log to me, which he started in the middle of March. He took these extensive notes because, he said, "things go in my head and shoot out the other side very quickly." The notes began with a department head meeting at the courthouse in March, with everyone scratching their heads and trying to figure out what to do that first week when schools shut down. The department heads started doing meetings twice a day—when they got to work and before they left, touching base with the hospital players first in person and then over Zoom. Matt also participated in calls with neighbors in Minnesota, including Nobles County, where Worthington is situated; he said, "since we butt up to the Minnesota region, it was great to actually hear what they were doing up there. They had some of the outbreak before we did."

"It sounds like they have been a bit stricter," I responded. I had just spoken to a nurse practitioner working in Minnesota who described how much better testing was there than Okoboji. In part because of the outbreak at the JBS pork processing plant, there was widespread testing and Nobles County reported more than 150 cases in May. She surmised that there were many more cases in the spring in

Dickinson County, too, perhaps because of the fluidity of people moving between these communities. She thought that they may have gone undetected because of the stricter testing protocol restrictions in Dickinson County that left most people out.

Matt continued, "They [in Minnesota] basically had a stay-at-home order in place for a while whereas our [governor] didn't do that. And, that's where you get into the politics. You can tell the Republican governors [like in Iowa] from the Democratic governors [like in Minnesota] mostly by which ones had the stay-at-home orders, and which ones didn't. So unfortunately, that's where politics were getting in the way of some things sometimes. I'm not getting into politics here, but you can definitely see that. But, yeah, they were shut down longer, and had more restrictions than Iowa did."

I asked, "Did you feel like there should have been more restrictions here?" I was curious in part because by the time I spoke to Matt at length (in late July), Nobles County's cases had dropped to a handful a week.

Matt continued, "You know, I don't know. I am kind of an opinion that the more you tell somebody not to do something, the more they are gonna wanna do it."

"It's like having a toddler." I chortled at my awkward mom-joke. I then raised my eyebrow as I thought about the ways people spoke about things like masking. I realized that people's reluctance to mask was sort of like a toddler according to social psychologist Erik Erikson. He argued that the second phase of psychosocial development—between eighteen months and two to three years old—focused on developing self-control. During this time the toddler grappled with the balance of autonomy and shame.[9] In many ways, American cultural squabbles about masking, which played out in real time in Okoboji, were not too far off from this dynamic. People wanted the *freedom* to unmask, while often wielding shame when anyone did the opposite of what they believed.

"Yeah, it is. You know, and it's kind of like the masking thing right now. There are people who will go out, they'll probably put one on if they have to. But by God if the government tells me I have to wear a mask, I'm not going to do it because they can't tell me what to do. It's that kind of attitude that is out there, with some people. And then they tend to be the most vocal ones, too. So that is what you get most of the time. Especially on social media, which I try to avoid. I haven't really been on Facebook for two years: that drives me nuts. But that seems like to be the kind of attitude that is out there."

"Have you had to deal with any community members who have been especially vocal, from your post?"

"There's been a couple who send like emails and letters and things. We had this public outreach committee going and making videos and posters and things. Maybe you saw some of that? We sent out a postcard: we pulled all of the property records of everybody that is outside the county that owns a property. Because we knew we would have a lot of people coming over the summer. So we sent out a postcard to say hey, you know, if you are going to come, quarantine at home for fourteen days when you get here. You know, stay home, stay safe.

"That sort of thing," he explained. "And we had one letter from a lady who said it made her feel very unwelcome and she didn't think that she was going to come this summer because of that postcard. And I didn't reply but I am thinking you must be the only one because things have been packed here since Memorial Day. And there's been a couple of letters from people in the public that, you know, [ask] why are you doing this? I mean they're citing different things."

"What are they citing?"

"You know, just things they hear on the news. Why are you opening the courthouse? And why aren't you doing this and that, and things like that."

Community queries like these waged on throughout the summer as the local response unfolded. Matt's experience introduces a core theme of this book: local officials faced community squabbles, social resistance, and cultural beliefs that made local-level management of public health recommendations hard. Some of this local-level resistance was deeply embedded in history, culture, and social relations. Let me step back a minute and give some context.

SETTLERS

People have lived around the Iowa Great Lakes Region since the last glacial periods (around eleven thousand years ago). Today, the Iowa Great Lakes Region encompasses seven lakes and six contingent towns bound together in

Dickinson County. The region includes Big Spirit Lake, the largest lake of the seven, which is surrounded by Spirit Lake, the largest town with around five thousand people, as well as Orleans, a small strip of lake and farmland. West Lake Okoboji is also a large body of water, surrounded by the small contingent towns of Okoboji (a Dakota word meaning "peaceful waters"), Wahpeton (a Dakota word meaning "people who live in the forest"), West Okoboji, and Arnolds Park.[10] East Lake Okoboji weaves between these two lakes and connects to West Lake by a strait covered by two large bridges. The towns around it are Spirit Lake, Okoboji, and Arnolds Park, which buttresses East and West Lakes. Three lakes weave off East Lake, including Upper Gar, Minnewashta, and Lower Gar. They flow into Mill Creek, which flows into the Little Sioux River, which flows ultimately into the Mississippi River. Finally, Center Lake sits squarely in the middle of the Lakes; most wetlands drain into Center Lake, where people quietly kayak and fish. Often people refer to this region as the Iowa Great Lakes and some just say Okoboji, meaning the entire region as opposed to the small town of eight hundred people.

Given the indigenous roots of the region, it is important to complicate the origin myth about when white families first occupied the Iowa Great Lakes region.[11] Okoboji was the summer residence of the Dakota people for centuries. The Dakota were historically eastern peoples, pushed westward. They followed the bison herds in the winter and lived around the lakes when summer came.

A small cabin in Arnolds Park has been reconstructed and become a popular tourist attraction that reinforces an

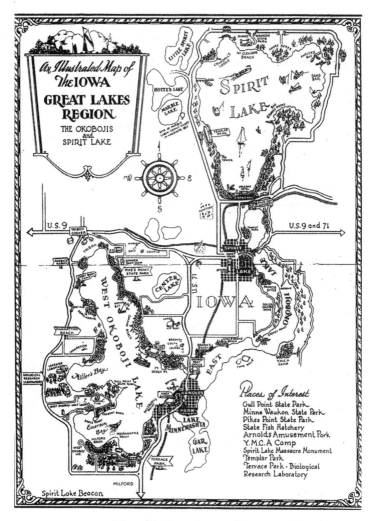

FIGURE 2.2. Map of the Iowa Great Lakes Region from the
Spirit Lake Beacon.

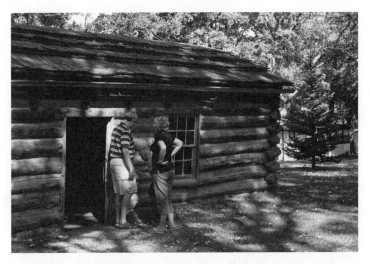

FIGURE 2.3. Abbie Gardner cabin. Courtesy of David Thoreson.

origin myth in Dickinson County. The origin myth of the community starts with forty settlers who traveled west by wagon to what was known as the Spirit Lake Region in late fall of 1856. They hailed God for allowing them to find rich fowl and fish and a beautiful lake.[12] These settlers were devout Protestants seeking a new life and land ownership. Each family claimed an acre or more of land and built a cabin. The claim to "free land" was embedded in the "American Dream," though the claim was only available to white European men who traveled west.[13] Like many others moving west, these settlers believed in Manifest Destiny, that the expansion of the US was both justified and inevitable. This was bolstered by the US government, which enabled white settlers to buy an acre of land for $1.25. Five million such acres of public land were taken from native populations and sold from 1854 to 1857 in Minnesota Territory.[14]

The Wahpekute Dakota returned home to the lake in March of 1857 after a hard winter. Their leader, Inkpaduta, led the small clan. Their pain was intensified by Inkpaduta's recent loss: his children, wife, and brother had been murdered by a white whiskey trader. Inkpaduta, now sixty, with smallpox scars visible on his face, was made a reticent leader. When the clan returned to the lake, they found their longtime home occupied by white settlers, claiming the land as their own. Inkpaduta's people were hungry.[15]

What ensued that spring is known by white people as the Spirit Lake Massacre of 1857. The historical accounts written by white settlers record that most of the original forty settlers were killed when the two groups met. But we know little about what actually happened. Public record suggests that Inkpaduta and accompanying Dakota men killed these settlers and took a thirteen-year-old girl, Abbie Gardner, as a prisoner. She was later traded for $3,000. Abbie went on to write her story, which was accepted as truth and memorialized in the restoration of her home and the cemetery where her family is buried.[16] Abbie's memoir is one of the "graphic, sensational accounts of killings carried out by the Dakota" that "whipped survivors, city dwellers, and politicians into a frenzy of revenge."[17]

After the conflict in Spirit Lake, the Homestead Act—signed by Abraham Lincoln in 1860—escalated the US-Dakota War. This decree gave a quarter of a square mile of land to every American citizen over twenty-one who could claim it. At this time, *citizen* meant white European man. In this way, it excluded the Dakota who had long lived on Okoboji's peaceful waters. Abbie Gardner, as a white woman, also could not own land. After fighting alongside Sitting Bull—the famous Dakota chief—in 1876 to defend Sioux lands in the Battle of Little Big Horn, Inkpaduta and his family left their beloved homeland and spent the rest of their lives in Canada.[18] Some descendants of these Dakota families reside today in South Dakota.[19]

After the conflict, the land was settled by soldiers from Fort Dodge and Fort Ridgley who came to investigate what happened in 1857. Many soldiers found the lake so beautiful that they returned and settled there after they left the military. Some stayed for generations, but many sold their land to businessmen who bought it cheap to promote tourism. The railroads were built in the 1880s and slowly people discovered the lakes and made increasing investments into land, steamships, and resorts. When the railroad company abandoned a planned expansion of the rails to Wahpeton on the west side of West Lake Okoboji, the investors planning a resort there tried to sell off the land quickly. My great-grandparents bought land cheaply from these early investors. The trains were vital as few people traveled by roads because the prairie was full of potholes and the roads would wash out in the rain.

Thereafter, northwest Iowa was settled by fiercely independent Dutch Reformists. In eastern Iowa, where a more collective culture exists, settlers were Norwegian; this is the area of the state that leans staunchly to the Left and has long made Iowa purple. (Although in recent elections, this area too has voted more conservatively.) In western Iowa, however, there is a rugged individualism that is reflected in conservative politics and values and that links back to the settler mentality. The community re-elected right-wing legislator Steve King nine times from 2003 to 2021, who the *Washington Post* referred to as "the Congressman most openly affiliated with white nationalism."[20] But the community is as Protestant as it is isolationist. One couple I interviewed for this project remembered stories of the Ku Klux Klan burning crosses on the Ocheyedan Mound in the 1930s to intimidate Catholic neighbors. There was a long presence of the Klan in the area, especially in Arnolds Park, because people distrusted Papists. Even today, people associate Democrats with Catholicism—although that's certainly not true for everyone.

Today residents of Dickinson County are largely white (96 percent) and the median income is around $58,000 per year, with 8 percent of the community living below the poverty line.[21] In comparison, its neighbor, Emmet County, is 87 percent white, 2 percent African American, and 8 percent Hispanic (mostly Mexican families who have now lived there a generation); people make about $10,000 less a year annually and 12 percent live in poverty.[22] Sixty miles south in Buena Vista County, median income is similar (around $54,000), but the resident demographics have changed over the past thirty years: 60 percent are white, 17 percent are Hispanic, 11 percent are Asian (mostly Hmong), and 3 percent are African American.[23] Storm Lake is situated in Buena Vista County, but despite the beautiful lake, it never became a tourist destination like Okoboji. Some people working in Dickinson County reside in these neighboring towns because summer jobs are plentiful at the Lakes while low-income housing is

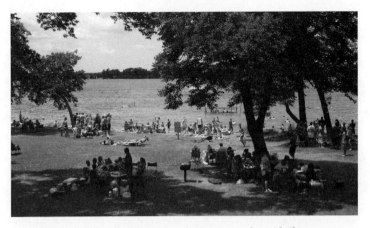

FIGURE 2.4. Pike's Point beach. Courtesy of David Thoreson.

in short supply, despite the constant building of middle-class homes.

I point out these demographics in part to suggest that terms used to describe America's Midwest like *heartland* and *Middle America* are political terms meant to white-wash a region that is in fact complex and ever-changing demographically.[24] Although the county in which I grew up, and which is the focus of this book, is mostly white, there is a history behind the homogeneity. Dickinson County has rejected plans to build a meat-packing plant to keep immigrants away.[25] In contrast, neighboring Emmet and Buena Vista Counties have embraced the agricultural industry, with significant environmental costs. Yet these communities have grown while other small rural Iowan towns have shrunk, and immigrant families have brought economic growth and cultural diversity to their communities (though not without social tension). They also have shifted these small towns closer to the political center. In contrast, Dickinson County remains very conservative, white, and Christian, with the large majority Protestant. Many of these families are linked to the original Dutch Reformist settlers in northwest Iowa. Today, immigrant families from around the region often travel for weekend trips in Okoboji: beaches are, at least on the weekends, frequently packed and increasingly diverse.

Midwestern historian Kristin Hoganson, from Illinois, argues in her book *The Heartland: An American History* that the idea of the heartland is based on a myth of whiteness that is "local, insular, and provincial" (xix) and even "isolationist," meaning "a desire to cut ties with the rest of the world" (132). Okoboji is not a "bubble," as many people I spoke to described it, where "rural Midwesterners [are] living on remote islands in the midst of the vast American landmass" (xxi). The concept of the heartland as epitomizing whiteness and settler mentality is in part based on, according to James Baldwin, the rejection of one's own ethnicity (such as Dutch, German, or Irish) and instead the acceptance of whiteness (which is in juxtaposition to Blackness and aligned with a belief of white supremacy).[26] He argues that the rejection of actual histories of genocide and enslavement cultivates a prioritization of "safety instead of life" and in doing so, white people "cannot allow themselves to be tormented by the suspicion that all men are brothers."[27] The idea of the bubble is inherently the rejection of anything non-white.

Historians have reinforced a myth of rural Midwestern communities, defining what has become known as the heartland as a moral concept.[28] This morality is based on a myth that "small-scale communities, church-centered social lives, family economies, and ties to place extending

over generations" are built upon the "stories of hellish
conditions inhabiting travel: mud, dust, mosquitoes,
assailants, unabridged rivers, dangerous forces, vermin-
ous lodgings, potholes, ice, snags, and paths that faded into
morasses of tall grass."[29] Frequently lost in this mythology
is the strong role of federal assistance in supporting farm
families in their pursuit of the American dream.[30]

This myth is exemplified by historical fiction such as
Laura Ingalls Wilder's famous series *Little House on the
Prairie.* In her Pulitzer prize–winning biography, historian
Caroline Fraser describes how Laura wrote the books to
convey what she perceived to be a "moral life" (250) based
on the ideals of her parents: "courage, self reliance, independence, integrity and helpfulness" (509). For example,
Fraser describes how the image of Laura's father, Charles
Ingalls, playing his fiddle around the fire and tilling the
fields, was of moral clarity. Yet her diaries and letters suggest elements of "moral ambiguity," often putting his family
in harm's way and relying on the government to protect
them while removing American "Indians from land he
wanted" (59). Many times, when the family faced hard
times, they hopped back in their wagon and regrouped
with family in Wisconsin before starting again, moving
between Kansas, Minnesota, Wisconsin, and the Dakotas.
In many ways, the family's constant moving reflected the
difficulty of homesteading, although often left out was the
truth of government support in providing subsidized land
and bailing them out when homesteading failed.

Fraser argues that Wilder's historical fiction constructed
a myth of self-reliance and antigovernment sentiment as

part of the American spirit. For nearly a century now the stories have been used by educators and librarians around the country to define what rural life was like. In the books and reconstructed sites for visitors, it is difficult to "distinguish between what belonged to the Ingalls family and what's a replica, between what is real and what is fiction" (514). Walnut Grove, one home of the Ingalls family, is only seventy miles from Okoboji. I visited a reconstructed site of the sod house as a child, wrapped in my bonnet and pioneer dress. We picked flowers and ran laughing over the sod house, thinking that we too could channel that history. My sister and I made cornbread, constructed teepees, drew maps of where they settled, and shook cream until we made butter.

MIDDLE GROUND

Moral ambiguities made many people wonder how seriously to take coronavirus. I spoke to a local metal worker (whom I will call Jay) who described himself as libertarian and an avid fan of the political podcaster Joe Rogan. Jay described how important the Facebook videos of Zach were for him in part because he was frustrated by the inconsistent messages conveyed by the national and state leadership. Jay was, however, reassured by the local public health leadership. My discussion with Jay revealed the tightrope many people walked between messaging around personal responsibility, wanting limited government in their lives, and wanting the pandemic to end.

Jay said, "I'm stuck in between a rock and a hard place because," he took a deep breath. "I'm trying to find the right words to use here so it's not just like . . . ," he paused again. "But like if this virus is that horrible and that deadly, why do I have to be tested to know that I have it? You know, if it's so bad! So those thoughts run through my head. Then ten minutes later I'm getting out of my vehicle to walk into Walmart and I'll put my mask on. Then again, I don't know."

I asked, "So you feel like, if it is that bad, we shouldn't need tests because you would just know that you have it?"

"Right," Jay replied. "And then again I know that it can lay basically dormant in your system and you're carrying it and you can have absolutely zero effects from it. But then you know, it could kill my grandma in days."

"Exactly," I said.

"You know, you get information like that and you're going back and forth and . . . ," Jay paused and looked up for a second. "It's just really hard and I think a lot of the reason it's hard for me is because of the political differences. Can you really trust anyone in our government to tell us the truth? So I just go by the hospital guidelines."

"Yeah."

"You know, I can't remember his name from Lakes Regional, he's on there all the time. You know, the one who looks like Lin-Manuel Miranda? Have you seen that?"

I burst out laughing. "Yeah, he's my brother-in-law."

"Well, he looks like Lin-Manuel Miranda and I swear to God one of these times I'll be watching a video and he's gonna break out and start singing *Hamilton!*"

Still giggling, I said, "Oh my God, can I tell him that? He would love that!"

"Yes, absolutely." Jay laughed right through his belly.

"You know, I love that because one reason I got involved is because I do public health stuff and he's been working on this so much. I've been trying to help out, you know? [. . .] But I don't think there is an easy solution. It feels just like all the stuff you're saying is dependent on a policy directive from the governor."

"Right," Jay said. "You know and then I was listening to our governor speak the other day at her press conference and, while watching her Facebook videos, I would read the comments. There were people begging for a shutdown and then the next comment would be someone saying, 'Don't you dare shut us down, we'll be just fine.' You know whatever. And it's like . . . ," he paused again. "They're so far apart, you know. 'I voted for you and I guarantee I'll vote you out because you won't shut our state down.' And then the other people are like, 'I didn't vote for you, and now I'm going to because you didn't shut our state down.'"

"And it feels so divided that it's not like there's a middle ground," I said.

But Jay disagreed. "There absolutely is middle ground but there is absolutely no way in my opinion for it to be reached because people have put up such big walls that there's just no way to even hear the other side."

IN-GROUPS

In 2020, two in every three people in Dickinson County voted for Donald Trump.[31] But people don't like talking about politics. A childhood friend who grew up attending the same Presbyterian church as my family said, "My mother told me never to talk about politics, religion, or your weight at the dinner table!" When coronavirus hit the area, partisan politics collided with traditions of propriety and politeness. This left the community conflicted about how to care for each other when everyday routines became imbued with political significance.

Social psychologist Jonathan Haidt argues in *The Righteous Mind* that there are six moral values that drive political divisions. These values emerge across contexts: care/harm, fairness/cheating, loyalty/betrayal, authority/subversion, sanctity/degradation, and liberty/oppression.[32] Haidt argues, "political parties and interest groups strive to make their concerns become current triggers of your moral modules. To get your vote, your money, or your time, they must activate at least one of your moral foundations" (156).

A good example of getting your vote through a moral value is by promoting the idea of caring. Caring is both innate and learned, and this is exemplified by caring for our young. Caring diverges somewhat when we move to political parties, sports teams, universities, and rock bands but maintains similar characteristics. Haidt says bumper stickers are the clearest in-group badges. Haidt provides two examples. On the one hand, a liberal "Save Darfur" sticker begs the reader to "protect innocent victims." The conservative "Wounded Warrior" sticker emphasizes those who have "sacrificed for the group" (157–58).

The loyalty construct was tested during the coronavirus crisis in 2020. I found that the idea of loyalty to the president became imbued in the mask debate. This can be understood by people not wanting "outsiders" (that is, liberals) to tell them what to do. In some ways, scientists were associated with liberals during the coronavirus response and therefore refuted by the right. The need to form groups is inherent in human history, where we have for centuries built "cohesive coalitions" to create a society we imagine (163).

This loyalty is exemplified by the strong alliances among those in Spirit Lake, Okoboji, and Harris-Lake Park School Districts who are particularly loyal to their local sports teams: the Indians, Pioneers, and Wolves. There have been repeated efforts (as with pro-sports teams) to change the Spirit Lake mascot from the Indians. For example, when I was student body president of Spirit Lake High School, we suggested changing the name from the Indians to the Muskies, which is a common and aggressive fish in the Iowa Great Lakes. (This name-switch was also suggested by our classmate, Tom Mueske, who was probably joking, but it stuck with us.) Yet there was strong opposition to changing the name because people's loyalties to what they know are intergenerational, social, and fierce. Moreover, for decades, some factions have suggested the three school districts merge to build a larger high school that can garner more courses, funding, and opportunities for student scholarship and extracurriculars. But many people fear such a convergence of groups will overshadow existing identities.

Similarly, there are strong alliances among those who cheer for the University of Iowa Hawkeyes versus the Iowa State University Cyclones. These loyalties are strong, unbreakable bonds. People become friends around these bonds and they are shared within extended families and across generations. Haidt argues, "Loyalty foundation is anything that tells you who is a team player and who is a traitor, particularly when your team is fighting with other teams. But because we love tribalism so much, we seek out ways to form groups and teams that can compete just for the fun of competing" (163). In some ways, the authority construct can be linked to loyalty when "people within a hierarchical order act in ways that negate or subvert that order, [and] we feel it instantly, even if we ourselves have not been directly harmed" (168). For example, people joke about marriages where one person is a Hawkeye fan and the other roots for the Cyclones. How do you survive football season?

These group factions were solidified further during the 2020 election cycle, which mirrored public health recommendations (like masking). When you wore a mask, you were going against the group. In many ways, people promoted in-group fidelity (that is, unmasking) through shame.[33]

Deep loyalties are particularly visible among extended families. Intergenerational households and communities are common around town. This means that many grandparents take care of grandchildren, or step in regularly. Many of my classmates have moved back or never left. They rely on their parents, have taken over the family business, or have started businesses with family. My family arrangements are similar. My sister moved her family back to the Iowa Great Lakes after spending ten years in upstate New York. She had left Okoboji to attend Bowdoin College in Maine and then spent several years learning about organic agricultural practices around the world. She now owns and operates a small organic livestock farm with considerable assistance from our father (a retired physician). My sister and Zach bought and moved into the house where we grew up, next door to my parents, who had done the same, moving into my late grandmother's home.

This is certainly not true for everyone. Many new families move to the area each year and this has significantly changed the local housing landscape. In high school, we ran a common cross-country route around Francis Sites, a neighborhood buttressed with farmland in Spirit Lake, that followed a sunny path of tall corn stalks in the summer. Today new communities filled with houses are there instead. The Lake offers a great deal to young families and has helped the community grow by attracting workers to rural businesses in northwest Iowa. Unemployment is the lowest in the state, but finding affordable housing in the region has been a problem for decades.

Haidt argues that some of these affinities are built through what he calls "moral capital" (338). This diverges somewhat from *social capital*, a common term in the social sciences. *Capital* refers to resources that enable people to procure goods and services. *Social capital* considers how social ties—among kin, neighbors, acquaintances, friends-of-friends—enable people to build trust and get ahead. *Moral capital*, in contrast, is the "degree to which a community possesses interlocking sets of values, virtues, norms, practices, identities, institutions, and technologies that mesh well with evolved psychological mechanisms and thereby enable the community to suppress or regulate selfishness and make cooperation possible" (341). While I feel this definition is somewhat overly deterministic, it emphasizes something I found in the Iowa Great Lakes Region when I returned as an anthropologist, as opposed to a summer visitor, in 2020. Moral capital, especially through language, loyalty, and conformity, is crucial for cultural bonds. In many ways, people used moral capital to collate support for backing a full return of the tourist economy as opposed to protecting the most vulnerable in town by prescribing to public health.

Moral capital is also aligned with the church. At least two-thirds of residents are active in a church—Lutheran, Presbyterian, Catholic, Episcopalian, Congregational, Evangelical, Methodist, and Baptist. There are also non-denominational churches that function like interdependent communities, relying on each other for money, faith, and familial support. Although each religious community differs in significant ways, it is a common belief that the church will lift you up (if you tithe and live by its moral codes). And in many ways moral capital does lift people up. Churchgoers tithe and give weekly offerings. Some of this money goes directly back into the community. For example, most social programs in the community are led by one church or a collection of many. There is a home for unwed mothers, a rehabilitation center for people recovering from substance use, food for indigent families. These are all led by local churches and demonstrate how loyalty and the values of protecting each other are central to local culture.

In many ways, what is conveyed as "faith"—meaning a devotion to God and community—is embedded in every-day talk. I am sure I spoke like this as a kid, embedding acknowledgment of the power I received from Him and

His Grace in my accomplishments. This way of speaking is not only learned in church. It is learned in school, the playground, and over coffee. It is communicated at work and in community spaces.

How people use faith in everyday talk reflects a central Protestant doctrine that faith alone, as opposed to work outside the self (such as in the community or nation) is enough to enter heaven. While Martin Luther's intention may have been for an individual to please God (as opposed to the self or society), how people engage with this doctrine today differs radically from that intent.[34] In many ways, a modern concept of identity grapples with how people perceive themselves versus how society sees them; it also requires them to negotiate their own personal needs and the needs of others, and to uphold the view that moral freedom is essential for individual dignity.[35] These essential tenets play into how many American conservatives see the world: "individuals should be allowed to get on with their private lives as they see fit. But freedom typically means more than being left alone by government: it means human agency, the ability to exercise a share of power through active participation in self-government."[36]

Speaking through faith, then, reflected a self-determination and rejection of authority that influenced people's resistance to masking, social distancing, and staying home. Instead, many people said, "I don't fear coronavirus because I believe in God," or "He will protect me." This use of language in many ways reflects an insider status, synergizing a strong faith, clear political position, and the confidence to go on with daily life without fear. Building a wide base of beliefs and speech through this faith was critical for the Iowa Great Lakes to open up Dickinson County and face the coming summer months.

CHAPTER 3

OPENING UP

IOWA WAS ONE of a handful of states that did not enact a formal "stay at home" order. Other states that instituted advisories without any mandates were Texas, New Mexico, and Utah.[1] Iowa was the last state to act, when Governor Reynolds closed schools, churches, restaurants, and many retailers for a few weeks. Many people mused, "We never really closed down in Dickinson County." With no lockdowns, many nonessential offices stayed open. From March to early May, there were only six cases in Dickinson County. As May approached, people started itching to get back to normal, especially when the sun came out and the lake warmed up.

State representative John Wills, speaker pro tempore in Iowa's Congress, wrote an op-ed in the *Dickinson County News* on April 28, 2020, titled, "When Should Iowa Reopen the Economy?"[2] He argued that "the vast majority of Iowans have remained healthy" and we must "be smart about reopening the economy." He suggested the state had reached the peak, or would in the coming weeks. He explained that he understood many Iowans feared opening up businesses too soon and spurring an outbreak. He juxtaposed this risk with the threat of financial ruin for many families if the county remained closed throughout the summer tourist season. Wills said, "Iowans can do both. We can fight COVID-19 by adding health precautions to protect ourselves and each other but also get people back to work and have Iowa thriving again." He went on to explain that Trump left decisions about reopening up to states. Governor Reynolds would soon reopen places like Dickinson County where cases and population density were low. He concluded, "There is no doubt that Iowa's best days lie ahead."

TOURISM

Representative Wills's comments about opening up cannot be dissociated from the powerful role of tourism in Okoboji's local economy. Tourism was central to my family's settling in the region, much like it has been for generations of other families who have lived in the Iowa Great Lakes region. People started coming to the lakes to fish, camp, and relax when the railroads were built through northwest Iowa in the 1880s. The Maritime Museum in Arnolds Park displays this history through a treasure trove of photos, memorabilia, old boats, swimsuits, tools, and even old amusement park rides. In that museum there are photos of my grandparents and Clements Beach Resort, which they ran for thirty years. For years there was a photo on the wall of the museum of my sister and I riding with Captain Kennedy during the maiden voyage of Queen II—

a reconstructed steam ship that still circles the lake throughout the summer. Captain Kennedy passed away a number of years ago, but many memories of his investment in the Lakes region continue on through the museum. For example, a few years ago a wooden slide built in the early 1900s for the old Fun House at Arnolds Park Amusement Park was restored and placed in the museum. Each summer I slide down it now with my kids, bringing back memories of my own childhood. The museum also shows photos from the early 1900s of tourists from Boston and New York standing beside human-sized paddlefish. These photos are astounding because current residents have never seen such exotic fish—tourists overfished them right out of the lake. There is a long history of locals and tourists exploiting the Iowa Great Lakes for riches. Most Iowans become rich because of farms. But in Okoboji, it's the lake.

Tourism has been used creatively by locals to promote the lakes, and there is no better example of this than the famous and fictitious University of Okoboji. Founded in 1978 (although the founders claim it dates back to 1878), the University of Okoboji was established by two brothers—Herman and Emil Richter, who run The Three Sons clothing store with their families.[3] The university was fake, but the founders used the ruse to sell the Iowa Great Lakes throughout the Midwest, attracting an increasing number of tourists and summer residents to the Lakes. The University of Okoboji is probably the greatest myth and advertising the lake has ever seen. The Three Sons, an upscale, outdoorsy clothing store in Milford, is itself a destination for tourists, in part because of the University of Okoboji

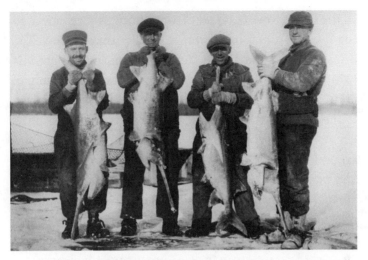

FIGURE 3.1. Okoboji tourists with paddlefish. Courtesy of the
Iowa Great Lakes Maritime Museum.

gear for sale there, and because it offers information about
the fictitious and undefeated Fighting Phantoms. While
most items price locals out, there is a packed sales room
upstairs. It is the place you go for a nice gift, a pair of shoes,
hiking pants, and a University of Okoboji sweatshirt, cup,
or blanket. There is always a Richter family member ready
to help you. The family is iconic at the Lakes. I grew up
with their kids and enjoy seeing my generation follow in
the Richter brothers' footsteps. In many ways, the family's
institutionalized status deepened with time.

Buy-in for the myth of the University of Okoboji is broad
and deep. The local radio station, KUOO, calls itself Campus Radio. The Three Sons store hosts the Winter Games
in January, a "homecoming" in July (topped off with a
marathon), and weekly summer events like soccer and

rugby tournaments. When I was young, we culminated the Winter Games by burning our Christmas trees on the thickly frozen lake while Herman managed the crowds. Now they burn trees on the greenspace and leadership of many local events such as the Winter Games has moved to the community. I too am invested in the myth, stuffing University of Okoboji trinkets into my suitcases to share around the world as thank you gifts for my hosts, friends, and mentors.

The investment in laissez faire living, in part through the rejection of serious study and embracing of play, was part of the University of Okoboji's legend. This jest is punctuated by a description on the University of Okoboji's website:

> Imagine a university whose founding fathers prescribed a curriculum fashioned not in academia, but celebration. An institution whose alumni promote get-down-and-boogie, not book worms. Such a lyceum exists only in mind and attitude, but it is steeped in a rich tradition in the vacation paradise of Northwest Iowa. The campus is the Iowa Great Lakes, and the halls of knowledge are the pathways of life. The University of Okoboji is a mythical, yet vibrant college of fun, spirit and goodwill.[4]

The tolerance of outsiders and loyal devotion to the local myth is further exemplified in the motto "In God We Trust. Everyone Else . . . Cash." In many ways, the emergence of this "University of Okoboji" myth, and its promulgation by locals and visitors alike, reveals how critical tourism is to the local economy.

The economic boom of the 1990s brought a great deal of wealth to the Iowa Great Lakes. People who invested in the stock market became richer. Newcomers dismantled century-old cottages and built ostentatious mansions facing the lake. Increasingly, new summer residents travelled by private jet, arriving on the landing strip across from my kids' favorite park. Tourists ate out, bought trinkets, and signed up for outdoor sports like parasailing and kite boarding. Some residents brought larger, louder boats to the lake. I remember one man from Sioux Falls, South Dakota, who flew to Okoboji after work to race his big, long, yellow boat from the northern to the southern shore of West Lake Okoboji. Then he got back into his private plane and flew home. Their noise was also a marker of change.

The 1990s was also a decade when families who lived in the region for generations left the lake. Although new summer residents flooded in, many families who had lived at the lakes were priced out by increasing home values and financial needs. These families sold cottages to investors because they needed the money. Families feuded when a parent or grandparent died and their cottage was divvied up by month, week, or year to their inheritors. Some children and grandchildren moved their lives elsewhere. Although there are still many century-old, multi-generational family cottages around the various lakes, most are dwarfed by their neighbors.

Slowly these mega-mansions shifted who could buy what and where. Outside interest in buying lakefront property, particularly in West Lake Okoboji, drove up property value as well as property taxes. It became difficult for people to justify a summer cottage, especially among those in the middle class who lived nearby, such as in Spencer, just thirty minutes south. It's nearly impossible now to afford a summer cottage. If you want to live on the lake, then you need to move there full time (unless you have money to burn).

With the influx of money into the lake, gaps between the rich and poor widened. There are clearer class divisions in the Iowa Great Lakes compared to other rural towns today and compared to my childhood. This wealth divide is in part because of the many industries that bring a bigger professional class to the community. It is also because of the very wealthy summer residents. But people come to the lakes from all walks of life: you don't need to have a lot of money to camp around Gull Point State Park, park an RV on Emerson Bay, and picnic at Mini-Wakan State Park on the shores of Big Spirit Lake. Locally there are a smaller professional class, a wide middle and working class, and a number of indigent families who struggle especially in the winter months.

One resident, who moved to the area to raise his family, explained the town clearly to me: "The vacation and tourist stuff gives this area a really interesting flavor in that a lot of towns the size of Spirit Lake in Iowa you are going to have people that just always live there. And here I would say it is a much more transitional population, even aside from the tourism, [due to] the ability to have some industries here and be able to bring people in. The idea of this as an area where people want to live, you know: they will get hundreds of applications for teaching jobs, and you know in Le Mars, Iowa, that is not going to be the case. And that is no knock on [Le Mars]. It is just in most of the places in this state, it is just a different experience. And then the vacation [homes], or the idea that there are multiple, and by multiple, dozens of million-dollar homes in a community this size is crazy. Or that each year there is some sense of who's got the newest boat and the nicest car, and just that all that lives in this area. The Iowa of my experience was people who had money and didn't need people to know it. The fact that they didn't want people to know, in fact that there wasn't the kind of outward to it that I think you see in this area. Now in fairness I think that is probably less true for the people that live here [year-round]. I think a lot of that is people who are seasonal, but it gives the area an interesting flavor. Now the benefit again, Emily, is not telling you anything that you don't know. But to have twenty restaurants and a seven-screen movie theatre, and three or four, five golf courses, and a summer theatre, and a YMCA in a community of fifteen thousand or ten thousand is ridiculous."

Many in town would attribute some of the notoriety and pull of the Iowa Great Lakes to a beloved public figure and local legend, Berkley Bedell. Berkley started putting together bait and tackle in 1937 when he was sixteen in Spirit Lake. According to the origin story of Berkley, his company, Bedell used $50 from selling newspapers to start selling hand-tied flies to fishing tackle shops and vacationing anglers. He worked in his bedroom, using clippings from his dog and backyard chickens in his crafty flies. The business slowly gained steam manufacturing an array of bait and tackle products and was eventually an enormous success, which Bedell attributed to "hard work, struggle, and tough times" that is "rooted in the idea of the American dream."[5] Most people who have fished in the past fifty years, at least in the US, have used a Berkley Trilene fishing line.

Berkley's son Tom Bedell ran the business after his father left to serve as a US representative for Iowa's Sixth District in 1974. Berkley was a Democrat and garnered extraordinary respect throughout the community, even with the strong conservative base.[6] When Berkley developed Lyme disease in 1987, he was frustrated that the Office of Alternative Medicine at the National Institutes of Health could not find a solution, so he founded the National Foundation of Alternative Medicine. In his memoir, Berkley says, "Time after time, in business, in politics, in my personal life, I have faced situations where it looked like there might not be any chance of success. But I found that by properly applying myself, I could overcome those odds."[7] When Tom retired, he sold Berkley, along with other companies he had acquired and named Pure Fishing, to Jarden, a large conglomerate of consumer brands, for $300 million cash.[8]

The influx of money into the Iowa Great Lakes in the 1990s also changed tourism. The days of family-run resorts where you return to the same cottage, friends, and resort owner's basement to sing over a vodka tonic were dwindling. My grandparents sold Clements Beach Resort to a developer in 1977, after running it for thirty years. Many other small family resorts shuttered their doors, with the

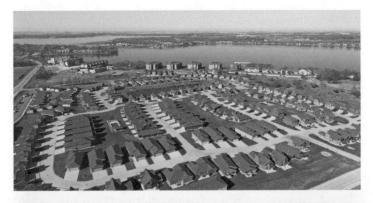

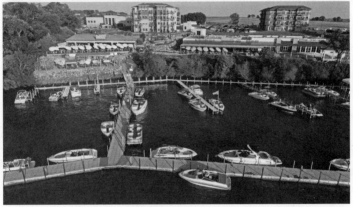

FIGURE 3.2. Bridges Bay Resort. Courtesy of David Thoreson.

exception of three: Fillenwarth, Triggs, and Pick's Resorts. But the loss of the small family resorts represented a bigger cultural shift when many people started to rent condos or private homes when they visited the Lakes rather than opting to camp.

The resorts that have been built in the past two decades are mega-hotels like Bridges Bay on East Lake Okoboji. Bridges Bay is both a resort and home. You can rent a hotel room for a couple nights, lease an apartment for the week, or buy a condo. You can buy a small patio home in the little village behind Bridges Bay, a community of part-time residents that replaced a rather sizeable farm. At the resort, there are two restaurants, both packed even on a week night. One restaurant is fine dining, but you can pick up a pizza there to take home any night of the week. The other feels like a beach-front bar, with fried food and fast drinks. There is a zipline, outdoor pool, and swim-up bar. They even have an indoor water park, which my family visits on rainy days or when the temperature dips below freezing. We rarely go there in the summer because the water park is swarming with tourists.

Developers also transformed the small quiet lakes of Upper Gar, Lower Gar, and Minnewashta into residential spaces. For decades these small lakes were preserved by Henderson Park, through which a windy and leafy biking trail runs, hugging the lake. This trail connects to the Greenbelt, which is miles of trails throughout the region and is part of the national rails-to-trails program. But developers have recently built big homes along their shores and advertised these homes as havens. These developers quietly served a crucial role in unbalancing the ecosystem of the lakes. While homes have always hugged Center Lake, half the lake has long been protected by conservation lands. During my childhood, the lakes were known for being quiet for fishing and kayaking; no big boats pushed you over there. But the three other lakes are no longer quiet, and the role these lakes played in balancing the ecosystem is shot.

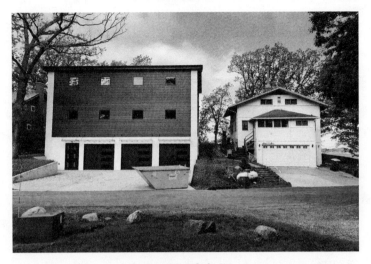

FIGURE 3.3. Development in Okoboji in 2020s versus 1970s.
Courtesy of David Thoreson.

This development reflects shifts in how people in the region see tourism. On the one hand, investors see money (at least in the summer months). Around seventeen thousand people reside in Dickinson County year-round, while more than one hundred thousand people reside there in the summer. Some weekends in July have reported up to half a million visitors. Most people visit Okoboji for a week or multiple weekends, mostly for boats, booze, and parties. In fact, party culture is so strong in the Iowa Great Lakes that everything is built around it: you can even buy drinks on the lake. This has become a source of conflict between families who have lived along the lakeshore for more than a century and those using the Lakes for profit. For example, when the biggest marina in town—Parks Marina—bought the Okoboji Boat Works (OBW) in 2001,

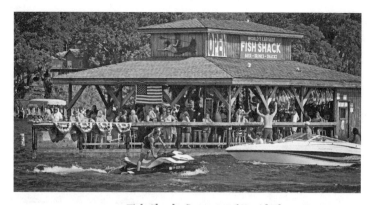

FIGURE 3.4. Fish Shack. Courtesy of David Thoreson.

the residents surrounding the boat works were up in arms because they thought the new venture would turn the quiet campus into a raging party of "karaoke, live music, hog roasting, and monthly full-moon parties."[9] When the alcohol license was blocked by the Iowa Supreme Court, Parks Marina's owner, Butch Parks, found a run-around and started selling liquor on a barge called the Fish House Lounge. It was parked on the lake outside the new bar and not under city jurisdiction because it floats.[10] He also started touring party barges around the lake—rain or shine.

Parks foresaw the tourist boom and planned for it. He bought large buildings two decades ago and encouraged people to store their boats in them. Now, you can live in Sioux City, buy a boat, store it at Parks Marina, and they will have it ready for you when you pull up in your car. They will also put it back in storage for the evening. Some of these boats are owned and others are rented. Over the past two decades, the intensification of boat rentals like these have contributed to bigger, faster, and more congested boat traffic on the lakes, infuriating locals.[11] For instance, when you rent a boat, you receive a map with a circle around Millers Bay so you can see where to tie up your boat to join a mass of boat-partiers on the lake. This traffic has had a significant ecological impact on the lakes in part because the marinas have so successfully promoted regional tourism.[12]

But after Labor Day nearly everything closes down. Most restaurants, bars, parks, and gift shops that hug the lakeshore find it's not financially viable to stay open after September. The resorts shutter their windows. Families leave to go back to school. International workers on J-1 and H-2B visas who ran the carousel and one-hundred-year-old roller coaster at Arnolds Park Amusement Park return home. People selling food, candy, or gifts return to their "winter jobs" (like working in the schools). Some visitors return for quiet weekends at the Lakes in September. Others make plans to return for the Winter Games.

A far-right Republican Iowan lawmaker who pushed to reopen the economy as soon as possible explained to me the complex intersection of tourism and coronavirus best: "It is complicated because our country is a culture that does not support the most vulnerable. And that includes poor people and that includes sick people. And so, like small businesses and businesses that rely on three months of income for twelve months of the year, you know, like we have no social safety net for those people. If they don't have some kind of a summer, we as a society, we as a culture say, well sorry! If you don't work, you don't eat."

The month of May signified a critical shift in how people thought about coronavirus in the Iowa Great Lakes. *Dickinson County News* reporter Seth Boyes wrote, "I was hopeful for a long time. I saw masks. Things were relatively quiet. But then the grind of cabin fever somehow usurped the reality of coronavirus, and our community seemed to shrug off the collective responsibility of protecting each other."[13] But it wasn't only cabin fever. The collective shift away from coronavirus was redirected toward keeping the economy afloat when business owners considered what a summer with coronavirus might mean for their bottom line.

Representative John Wills called to reopen the economy only a few days before Walleye Weekend on May 2–3, 2020. Walleye Weekend is the start of the tourist season, when people descend upon the Lakes from small towns and big cities to catch a number of tagged fish for cash prizes. In 2019, over 2,100 anglers from seventeen states descended on the Iowa Great Lakes for the weekend. The pot of prize money for those registered anglers who caught the first few tagged fish was set to $37,000; the most money was given to those anglers who could catch a tagged fish over the weekend. Most tagged fish weren't caught until much later.[14] The money generated from the weekend resulted in over $21,000 in donations for local water conservation projects.[15]

In 2020, the Iowa Great Lakes Area Chamber of Commerce cancelled the fishing competition planned for Walleye Weekend because of coronavirus. Instead, the Chamber extended the competition throughout the summer so people would not gather during the early days of the pandemic. But many people chose not to enter into the extended contest.[16] It was two weeks after the opening weekend that Tom from Sioux City caught the first tagged walleye and turned it in to Stan's Bait & Tackle; he wasn't registered for the extended contest so the $2,200 prize money per fish waited for the next person to catch a tagged walleye.[17] The money was never claimed.

Even though the start of the contest was delayed, few people cancelled their reservations for the holiday weekend and the hotels and restaurants filled with tourists. Many people I interviewed explained that they found tourist season opened earlier in 2020 because school was virtual. This was especially true for summer residents who arrived early to the Lakes to open up their cottages and settle into a place with low population density where it was easy to socially distance. But locals also described how they were shocked to see tourists descend upon the community before the governor officially eased restrictions.

On the Wednesday after Walleye Weekend, President Trump praised Governor Kim Reynolds as they sat together unmasked in the Oval Office. The president called Reynolds a "spectacular governor" who is "someone who has done very well in every respect."[18] The following Monday Reynolds loosened restrictions for counties with low coronavirus numbers, including Dickinson County. This plan was supported by an ambitious testing program that was described by state epidemiologist Dr. Caitlin Pedati at the White House. Vice President Mike Pence said Governor Reynolds was "leading the way" with her plans to reopen the economy and that "the outbreak in Iowa has not been like we've seen in other states." He continued complimenting the governor, saying, "It's a tribute to your early, strong steps."[19] When they returned to Des Moines, Reynolds and Pedati were notified that they should enter two weeks of quarantine after Pence's press secretary tested positive for coronavirus.[20]

By May 22, when their quarantine was up, Reynolds had reopened "movie theaters, zoos, aquariums, museums, [swimming pools,] and wedding reception venues" that had "appropriate public health measures in place."[21] This was the day before Memorial Day weekend. By the holiday, nearly everything in the state was essentially open.

MEMORIAL DAY

There were eight documented cases of COVID-19 in Dickinson County before Memorial Day. But that changed when the sun came out Friday afternoon. Tourists pulled up in their cars, towing their boats to slip into the lake. Those boats were full of gas and coolers packed with booze. The sun was shining. Ice cream was selling. The lake was buzzing. A long line of boats tied up together in Millers Bay. The restaurants were bustling. When night fell, the bars were packed.

Hundreds of people were infected with coronavirus in the Iowa Great Lakes as a result. With restricted testing, it's impossible to know how many people were actually infectious. A local twenty-one-year-old bartender at a popular and packed bar told me she was infected by a server in the week leading up to the Memorial Day weekend. She had symptoms by Friday. Her mother, a nurse at the local hospital, said it was probably just a cold. She served people booze throughout the weekend at the main bar, coughing, sweating, and taking Advil to ward off her headache. Three weeks later she took an antibody test and it came back positive.

Hank, a retiree residing in Arnolds Park, summed up the experience, saying, "For me there's a clear line up until Memorial Day. And, you know, at that time, as far as COVID is concerned, we—as I said we embraced the changes—we embraced the shutdowns." Hank smiled at me through the Zoom camera as we spoke in late June. During Memorial Day I was still in the DC area. I thought back on what we had been doing during the holiday weekend. I remember my family sneaking away early in the morning on Saturday for a long hike just an hour away from the city. I wrote in my journal that on Memorial Day itself my kids made cupcakes with our neighbor Hannah, who was part of our quaranteam. My eldest daughter learned a fiddle tune. My youngest slipped into the imaginary world that she had so frequently escaped to over the several months at home. We were itching to get to Okoboji, where their cousins were waiting.

"Was I concerned about numbers rising or getting ill?" Hank asked, flipping his head back and easing into his narrative. "At that time, no. No, I had hope that people would continue to behave like the grown-ups that we are. At least, the old, near-retirement-age people or post-retirement-age people that we would frequent these bars and restaurants with. Then Memorial Day came and . . . ," Hank looked down and shook his head.

I gulped, knowing where this was headed. I had heard an earful already from my parents, and it came up in every interview. What were people doing?

"What words should I use?" he asked as he continued to shake his head. "I guess *appalled, astounded.* I mean literally I would look at some of the people in the crowds, no masks, no social distancing. I heard the customers and some of the early reviews I saw of restaurants and bars. And, what the bleep is wrong with you people?" I smiled at his self-censorship.

"We had six cases here for two months," Hank said while he laughed uncomfortably. "You know? And now, as we, as you and I are conducting this interview, everything opened up and we now have 201 [cases] today and it's only going to go higher." Dickinson County was in the middle of an outbreak and cases had shot up from eight cases to more than two hundred in only a few weeks, raising the alarm of what this surge could mean for the community. Hank continued, "We all know who the major bar and restaurant offenders are in the area. It's not hard to figure out. All one has to do is drive by any of the local night spots after eight o'clock at night."

Most of the nightlife Hank was alluding to happens on Broadway Street (known as "the strip"). The first bar on the strip is Boji Nights Gentlemen's Club, which was for a long time the only place with a functioning ATM. Next door to the strip club is a pizza joint called Portside Pizza Pub. The bar opens up onto the sidewalk where people gather to savor pizza and guzzle beer from Coors Light to draughts of West O's Smoked Red and other craft beers from one of two local breweries. The same owner owns the next bar, Nautical, where people similarly mill around on the sidewalk or disappear into the back. Next is a huge wall supporting a three-story party palace, known as Captain's Getaway. Captain's can be impossible to enter after the sun goes down, in part because the bouncer at the door charges $50 or more to enter during the busy season. The owners of these two bars hold a great deal of social capital and political sway. For example, the owner of Captain's Getaway serves on Arnolds Park's city council. Both owners are big influencers in the Iowa Great Lakes Chamber of Commerce.

The next block is a combination of rib joints, dancing, refined dining, art, and coffee. The restaurant across the alleyway, Smokin' Jakes, serves ribs and other pub food and gets packed after midnight when the other bars close. People mill around just steps away at Murphy's, a bar capable of smushing hundreds of people together on the dance floor. Then the strip quiets down, with a family restaurant, wine bar, photo gallery, and coffee shop. Most of the other watering holes are sprinkled around the lake, miles from the strip.

This strip of night life is steps from the Arnolds Park Amusement Park (which mandated masks) and directly across from the century-old Emporium shopping center

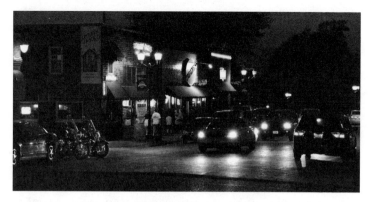

FIGURE 3.5. The strip on Broadway Street. Courtesy of David Thoreson.

(which didn't).[22] There were exceptions, however. The Sugar Shack—a small store tucked away in the Emporium that parents use to bribe their kids each summer—did require masks upon entry.

Hank continued, "The other day, my cousin Mike who lives in central Iowa wanted to know, 'how are things opening up in the Iowa Great Lakes?' I said, 'I will drive by and take a photo of Nautical for you.'"

I interjected, "Can you send me a photo?"

"I never made it and I'll tell you why," Hank continued. "The music coming out of there was so loud, I didn't even want to park my car. You know, if I'd had presence of mind, I would have used my Apple Watch and set it to the decibel meter. It had to have been way over one hundred decibels from out in the street. And it was packed. It had people spilling outside, everything." I smiled, thinking about how much fun it is to meet friends after sunset when my kids are tucked in bed; it had been months since I had left my house in the dark for anything but a late-night walk. I ruminated on how strange I found it that so many people were throwing caution to the wind. I had no idea places were so packed.

"And, you know," Hank explained, "their new business next door, Portside Pizza? It's pretty much the same thing. And I'll be happy to send you photos if you want. Pretty much the same thing. They've got a garage door that opens up at ground level and then they've got this lovely little perch with a bench along it. Um, yeah, it's . . . ," Hank paused and scratched his head. "Each one of those has six to eight people side by side with probably many dozens behind. No masks, no social distancing. I get it, they're there to have fun." Hank shook his head and tapped his desk with his hand.

"Who are the people that are there to have fun?" Hank asked rhetorically, and continued, "They're the very ones that are now coming down with COVID in that twenty-one to forty age group, primarily. You expand that up to the sixty age group and you've got, what is it, what did I just see? Two-thirds to three-quarters of our existing infections here. You know? The old people are smart enough in my view to stay away. Young people have decided they're over it. We're gonna have a good time. It's Okoboji, you know, like every other time."

Just after Memorial Day, on May 28, Debbie Parks—a co-owner of Parks Marina—was interviewed by local broadcaster Jeff Thee. Debbie sat at a table at the Barefoot Bar, wearing a blue tank top and sunglasses, with her hair blowing in the wind. "Everything changes when the sun starts to shine," she said with a smile and the carefree tone of summer. Behind her, you could see the square bar made of bamboo with servers and patrons sprinkled around it. Nobody was wearing a mask. "We know we need to be cautious, but we need to live. So, we're gonna move forward at Lake Okoboji and the Barefoot and all the marina district properties as best we can. And things are a little different, but we'll make it. And from the looks of last weekend, I'd say many people in the Midwest are ready to get out!"[23]

Jeff responded, "I think they are ready to rock and roll around here! I know boat sales have been good." Debbie described how difficult the spring was for the community and how everyone was in quarantine together. And she said, "We are still in this together," and "boating is a great social distancing activity." She looked at the camera and said thank you to everyone who bought a boat. Then she shifted to emphasize that the bar, restaurants, and gift shops were open for business. Now that the governor had lifted restrictions, they would return to business as usual.

Debbie joked, "I thought we were living in a real-life *Footloose* movie!" She meant that people found it difficult with no music or night life during the spring when everyone stayed home. Speaking about getting the musicians back on stage, Debbie said, "It's their livelihood. It's time to get these people back to work. They love to entertain. We welcome it! We welcome it! If you're ready to come out, come out. If you're not, I'm sorry. We'll try to service you from home, or curbside. So, baby steps. Everyone needs to make their own decisions."

At the time, many people were throwing around the excuse that "everyone had COVID!" in person and on

Facebook. This was in part meant to suggest you should forget your worries and get on with life—COVID wasn't that bad. But the older community members stayed home. Most elders in the Iowa Great Lakes region took coronavirus very seriously from the beginning. The gravity of concern they felt about the virus was directly tied to their personal risk of death or severe sickness. One retiree, who said her daily Bible study was the main thing keeping her sane, said, "we read things and listened to news and all that kinda stuff and got our masks on. Did we wear our masks right away? Yes. I think we did right away. I think I also started sewing the masks for the hospital right away."

Hank concluded, "And, that's all well and fine for [young people], but we all know that there's a catch to this whole thing. You know, I hope these people don't go home and go kiss grandma goodbye for their weekend visit because that might be it for grandma."

"And, anecdotally," Hank shifted in his chair and brought his head closer to the camera, like he was going to lower his voice and share something juicy, "and this is firmly in the realm of gossip, and should be treated as such. I have heard, not just verbally but also in a tweet forwarded around by six different people, about the number: forty employees of Parks Marina. And the whole Marina District, as they call it, coming down with COVID. And I don't know if that is true or false; those rumors persist." (Butch and Debbie Parks did not agree to interview requests for this book.)

"In my case," Hank continued, "I was never a really big user of the Barefoot Bar. You won't see me there. Not for a couple of years, probably, now. Even though for years,

I was a loyal tried and true customer of Butch Parks and Parks Marina. You know, I think they have a lot to offer, but in my view, if those are true, they are not respecting the community at all that I can see. And that's what it is for me. If you're a business owner, not only do you need to respect the community, but to continue your business, you need to earn the respect of your community. And some have been working hard to do that." Hank shook his head as he expressed his opinion.

Hank then shifted, "I was just telling some friends. I believe in giving credit where credit is due. When the Okoboji Store just opened, I would drive by, note the cars, note the crowds. When it first opened for the season, it was like "COVID, what COVID?" And then eventually I drove by and I saw there were fewer tables being occupied on the inside and also on the outside dining area where they roll down the shades. They were being spread out. Now I drive by, I see there's a process. You park in the parking lot. You check in with the hostess out front who is wearing a mask. They will find a seat for you either inside or outside according to your wishes. I think if you wish to see them sanitize it and hose it down, they will do that, hose it down, sanitize it and wipe it down in your presence. They will do that or they will go do it and then seat you. And you're seated by either a secondary hostess or a wait staff and they're also wearing masks. That tells me that they have some respect for their community and their customers. So props to them."

74

CHAPTER 4

OUTBREAK

I HAVE SPENT hundreds of hours of my life driving west on I-90. When I lived in Chicago during graduate school, I could drive home to the lake in less than eight hours. Once I made it in seven hours and fifteen minutes. Now that I live farther east, it takes at least eighteen hours driving west to reach Okoboji, mostly on I-90. It doesn't matter where I start driving. A piece of my soul releases when I cross the Mississippi River.

La Crosse. Saint Charles. Rochester. Albert Lea. Blue Earth. Fairmont. Jackson. That's where I take a left. I pass through a small town that looks lonelier than it did when I left. I see the turnoff to the Jackson County Fair. I pass the softball field I played in for years. My favorite ice cream spot closed and the building sits empty. I pass Fort Belmont, right where the speed limit increases. I put my foot on the accelerator and breathe in smells of cornfields and warm summer winds. I drink in the quiet and the stars. When I finally get to the sign that says "Iowa, Fields of Opportunity!" I know that I am nearly home. I then drive for fifteen minutes through empty fields where corn was just planted. I take a right at the drive-in theater. Fifteen more minutes and I slip into my parents' driveway, nearly always in the dark.

My family drove out to Okoboji on June 6, 2020, three months after lockdowns were instituted across the country. We had barely left our house since March, with the exception of escaping for long hikes outside of the city on the weekend. We were ready to see family and have a respite at the lake. Before we left, my husband, Adam, booked a $15 campsite at a small state park at the Illinois-Iowa border to rest during the drive west. But the morning we left I was so excited for an adventure that I woke everyone up at 4 a.m. and our campsite went unused. It might have been the sugar, the beef jerky, or the hundreds of songs we sang and bopped to on the way. But we made it by midnight.

The drive west was eye-opening. We drove through Maryland, Pennsylvania, and Ohio. When we stopped near the Indiana border, we noticed fewer people masking while filling up their cars. As we continued west, we saw even fewer masks. In some gas stations, you would never know we were in the middle of a pandemic. When my six-year-old had to get her wiggles out, we pulled into a gas station surrounded by cornfields and did cartwheels for fifteen minutes. My husband, Adam, filled the car with gas. When he came out of the gas station, he had beef jerky and a smirk. "They asked me where I was going and I told them Okoboji. They were like, 'you going to party there, bro?'" Adam laughed and shook his head. "I told them I wasn't planning on it. Nobody was wearing masks. We found the Wild West!"

The next morning everything felt lighter. We stayed with my parents but socially distanced from them, quarantining in the basement nook. The kids snuck next door to my sister's house and hugged their cousins. We hadn't seen anyone in months. The sun was shining. Lake smells wafted over my coffee. I was home.

Later that day I headed to Hy-Vee, a regional supermarket, to pick up a curbside order of groceries. I was aghast. Nobody was in masks. Not the person who brought my groceries. Not people in the parking lot. I spotted one person in a mask through the window checking out groceries. The previous week we had seen a police officer stand outside of a Wegmans supermarket in rural Maryland to ensure everyone who entered wore masks. It felt like a completely different world in Spirit Lake. Like there was no virus at all.

THE BUS INCIDENT

Cases shot up after Memorial Day weekend from less than five active cases to more than forty active cases. While this was small potatoes compared to surging outbreaks around the country, the instantaneous swell of cases alongside the start to the tourist season caused alarm in the public health and medical community. There were too few hospital beds to support a huge outbreak, and testing was still curtailed. In two more weeks, active cases had surpassed 150.

It was impossible for me to stand by and watch coronavirus spread throughout the community without trying to do something. The Fourth of July was coming quickly and many people worried that coronavirus would spread like wildfire across a prairie during the holiday weekend. I dove into interviewing as many people as possible to figure out who was getting infected, where, and why. When I probed, people opened up. I started piecing together the story and planned to write an article for the *Des Moines Register* or the *Sioux City Journal* that might shine a light on the growing risk of coronavirus infection at the Lakes.

I heard a rumor about "the bus incident" from Hank and others in bits and pieces at first. But it was not until "the bus" was referred to as common knowledge as the cause of the June spike that I realized how impactful it had been. My classmates who had teenage kids associated with the bus incident spoke about it with a subtle rage beneath their breath.

There were so many rumors flying around that it was hard to untangle fact from fiction at first. I thought back on Anne Lamott's expert advice in *Bird by Bird*, which Professor Annie Merrill had me read in college: take it day by day, slowly peel back the layers, and tell the truth.[1]

The more I talked to members of the community, the more people were willing to explain "the bus incident" to me in great detail. The most fired up and detailed was a classmate who I call Bethany, whose child worked at Parks Marina. She nearly jumped out of her seat when I asked her about young people getting infected. I didn't even mention the marina.

"Do you know when they first got it?" Bethany asked me. I had queried her about the June outbreak and why it was mostly young people at first. "There was a time when Parks

Marina, I don't know, had seventy-something employees positive at the same time. At the beginning of it, like around Memorial Day, Butch Parks, when he found out he had a couple of positive employees, he decided to put all his employees in some buses and bus them to Storm Lake, which was where the Test [Iowa] site was at that time. So they all could get tested."

At the time, the closest Test Iowa site was just sixty miles away in Storm Lake where there had been a recent outbreak at the Tyson pork plant.[2]

I scribbled down *70?* Everyone gave me a different number. I reached out to the Parkses to learn more about how they navigated coronavirus in their businesses amidst the pandemic, and possibly ask about the bus incident, but they declined to speak with me.

Bethany continued, "Well, if you have one person in any of those buses that takes an hour [and] twenty minutes to drive to Storm Lake, they are going to be positive. So, they all went down to get tested, I don't know how many were positive at that time but surely after that their entire staff was positive." I wrinkled my nose and scribbled down: *were all the staff infected on the bus?*

"Now the question would be: did he do that on purpose?" Bethany sat a bit straighter and said, "I don't know if he is smart enough to do that on purpose. But they were all positive shortly after Memorial Day, which is when Dickinson County spiked." I began piecing together—bit by bit—why so many people working in restaurants, from the kitchens to the dining rooms and bars, were sick at the same time.

One mom told me that she had heard there were out-breaks among the staff working in many of the businesses associated with Parks Marina, including their restaurants, Snappers and the Barefoot Bar. Her son cooked in one of the kitchens and got COVID-19 working without a mask because he said people were discouraged or mocked for wearing them. As a healthcare worker, she was concerned not only about her safety but also the safety of those she cared for. She also could not afford to lose wages. Before he was even infected, she barred him from staying in her house because she was worried that he might get infected at work. He was infected from or soon after the bus incident. After he recovered, she invited him to move back home.

It began to make sense to me why some people I spoke to suggested that there was a lesser strain of coronavirus in Okoboji. Some people jokingly called it "Corona Light." The puzzle started to come together. Cases were surging but nobody was dying because infections were circulating among young and healthy party people. I realized that it was perceived to be a lighter strain of the virus simply because youth were the most affected—with few having severe symptoms. And it became clear to me that the cause of this outbreak was party culture. So perhaps in some ways their interpretation of the social life of coronavirus was true.

"And then they were all healthy," Bethany continued, "and we had hardly anything with that group of people around the Fourth of July." I noticed her epidemiologi-cal sleuthing was beginning to make a lot of sense to me. People were sick in early June, and then immune by the Fourth of July. She went on, "So, you had no staff that was sick on the Fourth of July from Parks Marina. They had already been sick and recovered. So, was that on purpose? I don't know, like nobody was sick."

I began piecing together the June spike in COVID-19 cases with the bus incident, party culture, and mask-defiance. How many locals were involved in the June spike and who infected who? Where had people come from to party in Okoboji? Where did coronavirus travel once it left the Lakes? The hospital beds at Lakes Regional Healthcare were not full. But many physicians in small cities like Des Moines, Sioux City, Sioux Falls, and Omaha bemoaned the fact that these infections caused some tourists to end up in their emergency rooms. Those ERs were a long way from the bus.

Bethany shook her head, "Who puts them in a bus? Like you can't be in a bus together. But they all rode buses to the Test Iowa site."

She went on to explain that it was not only that the employer seemed to misunderstand transmission. He may have been trying to follow the rules and get everyone tested. It was the behavior of the young people that frustrated her.

Bethany explained, "There were some kids that, like a classmate, his mom posted [on Facebook] and said, 'Well, my son is another stat in Okoboji!' And I said, 'Oh, did you see that [he] was positive to COVID?' My daughter was like, 'Seriously? He is on my Snap story! He is in Millers Bay right now.' And I'm like, 'Well, his mom just posted that he is positive probably two or three days ago.' That means he then continued to go out [and party]! You know what I mean? He didn't care. They didn't care. They kept going out. They got tested and they would go bartend. And so here

I am telling my kid if you got [symptoms] and get tested, then you stay at home. But nobody else is doing that. That is what you are supposed to do. That is the right thing to do."

I found it so refreshing to hear my classmate, who was a vocal Trump supporter, describe quarantine as a moral decision. *It was the right thing to do.* In some ways, Bethany embodied the notion that personal responsibility was a serious task: that prevention was required of everyone. If everyone approached COVID-19 with the same care and caution as my classmate, then personal responsibility could work to stop the spread of the novel coronavirus.

"And I struggle with," she went on, "the discussion about mask or no mask. The people saying, my kids will never wear it!" Bethany shifted in her seat. I thought about how much sense this made because she was a healthcare worker. "I told my kids, here is the deal: you are not wearing a mask for yourself. You are wearing it for other people. And at the end of the day, you are never going to forgive yourself if you were sick with a stuffy nose or sore throat and you talked to the neighbor lady and she died two weeks later. Which I know that sounds morbid but the reality is that you are doing it to protect other people."

Bethany shook her head and sighed. "You can't teach adults to be compassionate or how to care for other people. That is what I struggle with."

COVID BAY

I was struggling with something else: Millers Bay. I heard people joke about "COVID Bay" around town. It was such a weird concept: that people were getting infected on the lake. But after I learned about the bus incident, I realized that the spike in cases happened among young people who cooked the food, served the drinks, and cleaned the tables at some restaurants and then would canoodle with those who worked at other restaurants around town. Eventually I figured out that it was on a certain day of the week when young people were partying together in the bay: Tuesday.

Tuesdays were considered "weekends" for young people staffing the restaurants around town because it was a common day off, meaning a particular group of people were partying at that time who were most likely infectious at that moment. This group of people contrasted somewhat from those who partied in Millers Bay on the weekends, which included young people and families and excluded many workers in restaurants and bars. One twenty-year-old summer intern told me, "I had two good friends who had a boat and we would go to Millers Bay. But no, we never went to Millers Bay on a Tuesday when everyone was there. I never went to like one of those." I asked for more details, and she continued, "people who work in Okoboji want to take Tuesday off and all go drink in Millers Bay, 'cause everyone has to work on weekends. So Tuesday is like our Saturday."

"I see, that is fun. But why did you not go on a Tuesday?" I asked as I slowly brushed away the cobwebs. Did the people on the bus infect their friends the following Tuesday? Is that how so many young people working in Okoboji were sick after Memorial Day? Were they sick from Covid Bay?

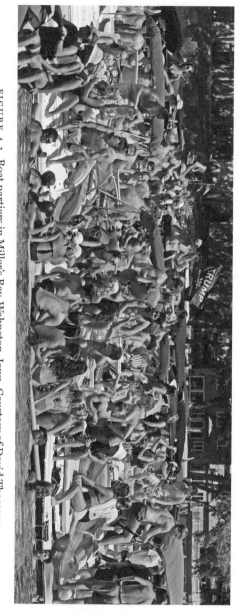

FIGURE 4.1. Boat partiers in Miller's Bay, Wahpeton, Iowa. Courtesy of David Thoreson.

"I was always at work," she responded. "One of the first weeks I saw someone's Snapchat story at Millers Bay. Everyone was dancing around a Trump 2020 flag. And I thought, no that is really not my move, not the people I want to hang out with. But also, like there were things they were talking about when we were trying to make decisions about what we should do. There was this older lady that we worked with, she was just the nicest that she could be, and [my roommates and I] talked about how, if we got coronavirus and we gave it to her, we could like seriously change her life. Like, you know, she could die. And there would be a guilty conscience on our part. So that is why I didn't participate in that kind of stuff."

Other young people I spoke to were more flippant about partying in Millers Bay. "I've been to Millers plenty of times this summer," a bartender told me. "Whether I'm with my family, or tying up with my family or friends, or with my friend tying up with people our age, it seems to be pretty normal and no one is really caring. But it is so different here. Like I would put a Snapchat story on and be like this is right now! I'm like, yeah, this is right now! I think it is young people wanting to have a normal summer and go out and do everything. But from what I've heard, a lot of people my age have gotten it."

I asked her if her friends were getting tested. I was so curious about how true the numbers were. I had a hunch that the actual numbers of cases in Okoboji were much higher in June than the hospital reported through testing.

"One of my guy friends had symptoms and he went and got tested and he was positive. And then his guy friends were like, 'we don't have symptoms but we should get tested just to make sure, then we might not have to go to work!' I think they just wanted to not have to go to work but like five of them had tested positive even though they had no symptoms."

I scribbled down: *how could we ever know how many young people had it but never had any symptoms?* Coronavirus was so baffling in part because of this unique characteristic: people could get it, carry it, and pass it on to others without ever knowing. The young bartender added, "There are so many more people that don't know they have it."

Millers Bay carries multiple meanings for me. Five generations of my family have grown up on West Lake Okoboji, starting with my great-grandparents. They bought the property in 1907—the same year they completed medical school in Des Moines, Iowa—and spent most summers at what would become known as Clements Beach. They instilled an unwavering love of the lake in my grandfather. He took the multiple cabins my great-grandmother's family built over several decades and started Clements Beach Resort. My dad grew up there, and, even though it was sold five years before I was born, my family lore resides there. Sometimes when I stand on Clements Beach and look across the waves, I think about my great-grandparents paddling their small boat across the lake for provisions in Arnolds Park three times a week. I think about my grandparents repairing, painting, and cleaning cobwebs from cabins year after year, preparing for new visitors. I think of my father tromping through Little Millers Bay, checking his traps that remained empty as the sun rose in the

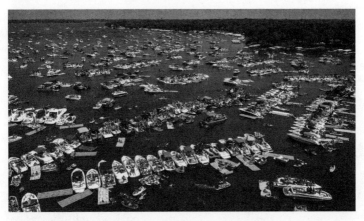

FIGURE 4.2. Aerial view of "COVID Bay." Courtesy of David Thoreson.

east. Years later he taught young people how to waterski in front of the resort. I would wakeboard with my friends in the same place a generation later. But now it's much too congested, unless you get there at sunrise.

When my family settled in Millers Bay, a century ago, a small part of the bay was an estuary that was so shallow and mucky that nobody would build there. This is one reason the state set up the Lakeside Laboratory there to study the fish, algae, and water—just a hop, skip, and a jump from my family's property.[3] I have used "the lab" as a summer writing oasis for years, sneaking into the Limno Lab—settling into a rickety desk adjacent to an empty basin that was once full of fish, crayfish, and turtles—to find some peace and quiet. Other times I lurk in the library at the Lakeside Lab, where I am only disturbed by my husband working nearby and looking for snacks.

But now, because of heavy traffic, the laboratory is studying how recreation is harming the lake. Boat anchors have torn up the lake bed and disrupted aquatic foods. The toxicity of garbage and feces is killing the fishes' breeding grounds.

This intense recreation is one reason that many people considered Millers Bay more infectious in June 2020 than anywhere else in the area, because so many people were convening there, mixing fluids and fomites. It became a hotspot that drew national attention and infected many young people in town.[4] At least one death was rumored to be directly tied to Millers Bay.

One of my earliest conversations with a bartender gave me some context about what young people were thinking when they tied their boats together in Millers Bay. The young woman I spoke with said, "Most people getting sick and obviously spreading it are people my age. And that is because of the bars and because of, I think, Millers Bay. People like to hang out on the boats and then you have a ton of people on the string of boats. And people are two feet from your face and you're getting past people always. It's just all the time. So I think the big, big reason [coronavirus is spreading] is the bars and boats." I looked down at my notebook and drew diagrams to make sense of where people were getting infected, and where those people were then infecting people. The bars and boats made sense.

She then reflected, "And so, I guess I don't know. I feel like we're not spreading it really through the restaurant business. Again, I don't think other restaurants really are either." I listened intently here because I thought she was trying to tell me that she did not think patrons were getting sick from dining in the restaurants young people were working in. This was a huge concern for the local economy: that the restaurant business would slow.

She concluded, "I mean, it's the bars. Because the bars don't really give a shit about social distancing. It's just packed."

"So, you feel like late night is kind of when it's being [transmitted]?" I asked.

"Yeah, and my bosses don't really want me to go there [to the bars late at night] because, not to sound like on my high horse, but they really need me behind the bar."

CHAPTER 5

BUSINESS AS USUAL

AS THE COVID cases ticked upward in Okoboji, I saw a classmate post on Facebook that he had gotten coronavirus in the bars around town. He had become a successful tradesman and is well respected in the community. An outspoken Trump supporter, he is very open and proud of his conservative politics. Frequently on his Facebook page there are references to God and Country, support for Blue Lives Matter, pro-life rhetoric, and jokes about Democrats. I do not think his views vary much from the majority of locals in the Iowa Great Lakes region. I followed his Facebook feed throughout the summer because his views captured for me the essence of culture and belief in the area when he reposted the following message to his Facebook page: "They're telling me the virus is everywhere. I told them so is God. Can I get an Amen?"

I pondered his post and wondered if something bigger was happening. I reached out to more classmates and friends to figure out not only what was driving infections but also to understand differences in how people in Okoboji thought about coronavirus and the ways many people in my professional circles were thinking about it. I knew the increase in cases was not only the fault of young people who were on the bus and then partying in Millers Bay. Was it cultural? Social? Linked to profit?

Midwestern states were slow to see coronavirus spread into their communities. Seattle and New York City faced alarming outbreaks at the beginning of the pandemic in part because of their density and because weeks passed before people realized the virus was circulating. By the time people realized how much virus had circulated throughout the cities, the hospitals were filled to capacity and fear was seeping through the veins of the nation. But with so few cases for so long in Okoboji, many people thought they had dodged a bullet. Was the worst over?

A local public health official whom I will call Dave explained their thinking in those early days of the pandemic: "We don't wanna say the sky is falling before it truly does here. Like yes, in New York and out East it hit very very bad and we were still yet to see very much at least in Iowa. And for better or worse we held off on saying stuff for a little while. It was more planning for what should the hospital be doing: how can the hospital be prepared? And kicking that into a high gear to make sure we were prepared and ready to go."

Dave continued, "I'd say the conversations were about how were we going to communicate about people staying home, social isolation, and trying to push stuff out to the businesses. And I had a lot of the communication channels set up and open through different stuff for Public Health and—getting their messaging out. And our big push was to figure out where is the good information coming from? Because everything was changing so quickly. So rather than us staying specific, 'You need to be home for fourteen days, do this, do that,' we were really focusing on, 'Hey there's a lot of noise out there. You want to listen to the CDC, the World Health Organization, or the Iowa Department of Public Health. This is what you want to be taking, these are current links for that.' That was mainly our message in the beginning. And at the hospital I know people were getting annoyed because we'd come out with a policy on Friday and we'd meet Monday and say, 'Well, we need to change that again,' and send something else out later today. And it was one thing to do that with the hospital, it was another thing to do that with the community."

"And how do you think people responded?" I asked.

"Surprisingly at least when we first started, a lot of that messaging was, 'These are your good sources, this is closing down, this is some of what it means.' People were very responsive at least at the very beginning. And they seemed to take it to heart. They called us if they had any questions or concerns, and it worked very well at the beginning."

Later I heard more from the public health team about fielding community questions. Like all small towns, neighbors ratted out neighbors, and community surveillance became status quo. One public health worker said the calls they got were so funny, like "Karen down the street is coughing on my tomatoes."

Dave went on, "Internally, you have the people that say, 'Oh it's still a hoax', all the way to the people that say, 'Oh my gosh, someone's infected in Des Moines, what are we going to do here?'" Dave paused and thought for a minute. "Which it probably was already here then, we just couldn't test. Kinda the whole gambit, the whole spectrum of people not caring to people caring probably too much at the beginning."

"Do people in the hospital think it's a hoax?" I probed this way because I had just spoken with a nurse who was up in arms because her colleagues were posting pictures on Facebook of themselves drinking at bars, dancing up close to tourists, sharing drinks, and smushing their faces together for selfies. This behavior was exactly the opposite of what Bethany, also a health practitioner, had described as personal responsibility to keep the most vulnerable safe. "And in a pandemic!" the nurse said, infuriated that they might bring the virus into the hospital.

Dave continued, "I guess hoax is taking it a little too extreme. It's just 'Eh, everyone's gonna get it, whatever, herd immunity.' But way more laissez-faire. It's concerning because we still wanna protect ourselves and do what we can. Surprisingly yes, there's people in the hospital. I'm sure Dr. Borus, maybe in a closed conversation, would say that even within their own provider group they have the whole spectrum of people that are almost to the point of way overboard to the point of 'Whatever, I'm not wearing a mask, I'll go to the bars, who cares.'"

"Why do you think people feel that way and do that?" I queried, as I scribbled down, *there are doctors not taking coronavirus seriously in town?* At the time, I found this truly shocking, that medical professionals—a family physician, nurses working the emergency room—were not only dismissing the risk of coronavirus but potentially working to undermine efforts by Zach and others on the public health team to mitigate infections.

"I've had this conversation with [others] and it's . . . , I don't know. I've been doing the cop-out One-Third Rule: anything that you say, a third of the people are going to love it, a third of the people don't care, and a third of the people are gonna hate it. I wanna say some people have to push back just because you told them to do something, and I don't know where that comes from. It's quite irritating, too, because we've switched a lot of our messaging to 'You're not doing this for yourself. You're not protecting yourself. You're doing this for others around you.'"

I heard in his voice how frustrating it was that his whole campaign was focused on *getting people to care about others.* With a county, state, or national mandate, his frustrations would vanish. The local COVID-19 task force knew this. Zach and the hospital repeatedly urged Governor Reynolds for a mask mandate or other public health leadership from the state level. In fact, when Senator Joni Ernst visited the local hospital in June, Zach described the situation of rising COVID-19 cases and reasons to take more stringent public health measures.[1] He recalls that Ernst thanked him for his input and then jokingly called him a "Debbie Downer," swiftly moving the conversation ahead. The public health team also lobbied the County Supervisors throughout the summer to enact and enforce a mask mandate locally. The County Supervisors refused.

A local lawyer told me that he had heard the sheriff state in public on multiple occasions that he would never enforce a mask mandate. The lawyer told me that he believed the governor felt the same way: "I think that part of it is that the governor recognizes that she can say things like 'We are supposed to be doing this,' or 'I highly encourage Iowa to do the right thing.' But I think the reason she doesn't make it mandatory is because I think she is recognizing that unless you are actually going to put your money where your mouth is, and enforce it by rule of law and all of that, I think she knows it is stupid. I think she doesn't think that is practical."

Dave explained how frustrating it was when people could not "get on board like a lot of the other countries have been doing with masks, even a lot of other regions of America are doing." He mused, "it's too bad people don't listen more often and take it to heart."

"But why?" I frowned, thinking about how different it was in the Washington, DC, region, where people would shame you for not wearing a mask. Shame was a powerful tool that was wielded in wildly different ways.

"Yeah. I go to the YMCA every morning," Dave continued. "And I'm the only one that wears a mask my entire workout. And this is subjective, but I work out infinitely harder than anybody else there, and I can somehow still breathe with my mask on despite . . ." Dave laughed, and I laughed too. He sounded like Adam, who is an athlete and can't figure out why I want to stick to my three-mile runs as opposed to his marathons. Dave now spoke with a smirk: "I make it through. I don't know what the big issue is."

"We get a lot of questions from staff members and task force members saying, 'It's so uncomfortable. It's so annoying.' Okay? So is sitting in the ER. So is [hiring] extra staffing for a hospital and still not having anybody in the hospital. There's a lot of things that are annoying in this world and this is a very minor nuisance. And those are the ones that just make me growl at home, 'cause even some of my wife's friends. There's some families that are like, 'We have not gone anywhere. We've not done anything.' And there are some that are like, 'Whatever.'"

"I think people have this blockage or a wall. They're like, 'I just don't want to do it, I'm just not doing it.' I don't know." Dave's reflection made me think of a commentary written by medical anthropologists Lenore Manderson and Susan Levine early on in the pandemic; they spoke of a powerful link between white privilege and the urge to get on with life, despite risk to others in the community.[2] I could not help but wonder what makes people in Okoboji—or pockets of America—think they are so exceptional compared to the rest of the country.

"I don't either," Dave said. "I feel a lot of it is peer pressure. Maybe that, or the people they look up to aren't doing it."

BUSINESS DECISIONS

I shifted course to ask Dave about his interactions with the Iowa Great Lakes Chamber of Commerce. I had quickly realized how powerful they were in directing how businesses should (or shouldn't) respond to public health recommendations. First, I had asked my father, a city council member in Okoboji, a town of eight hundred-ish people, why they did not shut down businesses. He looked at me thoughtfully and said, "I'm not sure. I'll bring it up with city council." He emailed his fellow council members and received a tepid response. He eventually said, "I think people see the Okoboji City Council acting alone, without acting with the adjacent towns, as inefficient. If Okoboji City Council mandates masks or enforces social distancing, then people won't visit the few restaurants in Okoboji. They will go to Arnolds Park. It has to come from the county supervisors so everyone is affected equally." I accepted this explanation in part because the owner of a large family-run marina and restaurant was on Okoboji's city council. Similarly, the owner of the busiest bar on Broadway Street was on Arnolds Parks' city council. Business interests were everywhere.

I asked Dave, "Did you have any interaction with the Chamber of Commerce?"

"They are very . . . ," Dave paused and looked up at the ceiling as he thought carefully about his next words, ". . . very hands off and we've even had the chamber president call our CEO [at the hospital] because someone was giving pushback saying, 'Why is the hospital requiring everybody to wear masks?' And was getting upset over why we kept putting [public health] messaging out there. About that point, the chamber's CEO said, 'Hey this is what I'm hearing!'"

I paused, and scribbled down: *The director of the Chamber of Commerce called the hospital's CEO and asked them to stop educating the public about coronavirus. What?*

Dave went on, "Comparing it to some other chambers like the Spencer one, for instance, they're very active." I wasn't surprised to hear the public health department in Clay County, where Spencer is, was active and engaged with

97

the business community. Spencer was thirty miles away but had minimal tourist industry, although they did host the nation's biggest county fair every September (which they cancelled in 2020).[3] "So, Clay County is very active in putting out information to encourage masking and to help with that and sharing information and pictures of people wearing masks and doing that. And same with, I want to say Dubuque or somewhere else. They put together an entire tool kit for the community of, 'Here's how you can open safely.' And our chamber's not wanted to bite at any of that and not wanted to touch that with a ten-foot pole."

"I'd hate to politicize it any more than others, but . . . ," Dave paused for a minute, ". . . and I'd say I probably lean more to the right, as well, which is what makes it even more annoying. There's a lot of very strong businesses that are incredibly Republican, incredibly to the right. Whether or not this is a factor, I'm guessing they're pushing a lot of that like, 'You don't get to say that!' Or, 'I'm going to pull my funding back. And I own twelve businesses here so good luck. We'll drop out of the chamber, all twelve of us, and that's going to decimate your funding.'"

"So there's a couple actors you think who are pulling the strings or leading?" I probed.

"That would be my guess. And going from where a lot of the infections have been coming from and where, basically they're not gonna come out and say anything like that. Anything toward the lines of, 'This is what we're doing to protect you. You should be masking and my staff are masking.' Those places are very not [requiring people to wear masks]! And they're walking the fine line of, 'Oh! You said 50 percent capacity: All right we'll be right at 50 percent, barely follow the rules.'" He finished with an awkward chuckle.

Dave gave the owners of Parks Marina as one such example in Okoboji. For instance, they are a conglomerate of eight businesses. An employee for the marina conglomerate sits on the board of directors of the Iowa Restaurant Association Board.[4] I heard many people suggest the owners can speed dial the governor any time to request that something change in their favor. They are also politically connected in the Iowa Republican party, donating a great deal of money to longtime right-wing representative Steve King.[5] "And they don't have any masking and they don't encourage their staff to," Dave said. "I would say they've done a good job of making sure their staff don't return to work when it's reported. But, no masking, no requirements."

"I interviewed a girl last week who works for them," I said. "She said she was forced to go to work after seven days even though she was told [by public health] to stay home ten days. They made her work. Isn't that illegal?" In fact, as the summer wound on, I spoke to three young people who worked for the Parkses and described allegedly precarious working conditions, making them feel unsafe. Two said they quit and one said she finished working through the summer because she needed the money and felt she had no other choice.

"Yeah, I would say they're a huge driving force. And Butch Parks was never one to mince words and I wouldn't doubt it one bit. This is all conjecture and guessing on my part that he's probably saying, 'You don't say anything about masking. I'm not doing it and I'll pull out of the chamber with like eight businesses!'" I listened intently, unsure if he would really say that, or if he would pull out of the Chamber of Commerce. But this statement underscored the type of respect and power he wielded within the local economy.

"So, it comes down to money," I repeated. "And it comes down to who gives fees, donates, who pays membership fees? I hadn't really thought about that, that is so interesting."

"It's very annoying that the Chamber has not been reached out to for anything. I know [the hospital CEO] is on the chamber board and I don't believe they've asked his input or insight for anything. It's just, 'Whatever, we're just going to continue as normal and put out information about our businesses like we normally would.'"

I wasn't very surprised that, even when the head of the hospital was on the board, his expertise was apparently not sought. Science was largely sidelined in the business industry in the Iowa Great Lakes. But not everyone was like that. The office of public health and the hospital had encouraged Zach to do a couple of virtual meetings for the business community as the summer marched on. Many people were courteous and some appeared amenable. I spoke to my high school prom date who was on the chamber board and taking COVID-19 very seriously. He worked with his father who was high risk. Yet whenever I asked him direct questions about other businesses, or the board more generally, he shook his head. Clearly, people had different views, concerns, and priorities, even in the business community.

Dave continued, "At least in the state of Iowa you're really not breaking any laws. Kim Reynolds has been very clear like, 'We're hands-off. People can do anything they want.' Which has been very annoying. When people call in, we have been very careful to say, 'This is our recommendation. We can't force you to do anything. This is our *recommendation!*'" This made me think about a headline I had seen days before in the *Des Moines Register* that gave me pause: "COVID-19 Response Should Protect Working Communities. Why Is the Governor Putting Corporate Profits First?"[6]

I spoke to many locals, however, who were hesitant to visit restaurants that blatantly ignored public health recommendations. A guy pushing thirty (who I call Jeff) told me, "Maybe it is wrong but I generally don't know if I will go back to a Butch store again." Jeff meant a store linked to the Parks Marina conglomerate. He felt like he faced a moral quandary.

"Tell me about that?" I asked.

"This was before things even spiked here," Jeff explained. "We were cooking nonstop but we thought we should support the local restaurants. It doesn't mean we had to go to a restaurant, even though they were only open 50 percent capacity. We tried to order takeout and kept getting busy signals when calling the store. So Barefoot Bar was right down the street, and I thought I'll just drive over. And I was very disappointed to see that like, I wasn't counting heads, but it was more than 50 percent capacity in there."

"When was this?" I asked.

"This was late May," Jeff said. "I've gone in there and taken pictures. Maybe they changed things later."

"Well, they just got fined," I said, pointing to their violation of Governor Reynolds's crowd restrictions as the summer waged on. This had such a big impact that they seemed to have closed down their crowdcam at the Barefoot Bar (a constant stream of video footage of the ongoing parties at the bar).[7] The *Dickinson County News* stated, "State officials said the Barefoot Bar on East Lake Okoboji did not ensure its patrons were separated by at least 6 feet of distance, failed to limit individuals from congregating and failed to implement reasonable measures for increased hygiene practices."[8] They were fined $1,000.

"It was crazy busy. It was the Tuesday right after Memorial Day," Jeff continued. "But they were packed at lunch and then at dinner time they were all the way shut down. And they were shut down all the next day. So, it was like, 'Oh?' But we went later and I said, 'Why don't you order takeout?' They said, 'Oh we can't do take out right now, we are too busy.' And I said, 'Well that doesn't go well for your 50 percent capacity.' And I said, 'Why are you not doing takeout?' And they said, 'We want people to come here and enjoy the view.' And I said, 'I don't know, it seems to incentivize poor behavior to me.'"

"Interesting," I quipped. The bar is well known for being a laid-back place to party, where you can also bring your kids to climb on the jungle gym and play in the sand.

"I just felt that if you are trying to push poor behavior, then people can come. You are not trying to even give people the option to make the choices, so that really upset me. It rubbed me the wrong way." Jeff continued, "That tells me as a business model, they make all their money on alcohol. That is why you want someone coming into your restaurant. Because alcohol is your biggest money maker. And if people are doing takeout, then you are probably not taking money from alcohol."

At the end of my interview with Dave, who was completely consumed with the public effort, I asked, "Do you think it would've been a different summer if people were required to do certain things?"

"I think so," he replied. "Whether or not that would have changed a lot of the stuff that's happening here? I'm sure you saw the pictures of Millers Bay. Or just driving around on the weekend heading back from wherever. I would say yes and I think there's evidence to suggest yes it would be different when you look at a lot of other communities."

MODELING

A few days later—still in the middle of June—I asked a local community leader, Tara, how to promote public health before the holiday weekend that was fast approaching. Should Zach pen something for the Chamber of Commerce newsletter? Tara said, "Zach's been making a statement over and over again. The people that listen to Zach are already listening to Zach."

Tara quickly pivoted and spoke rhetorically, "Can you get the chamber director to do it?" I could tell she was not necessarily asking a question but rather making a point that, in her opinion, the head of the local Chamber of Commerce would not support the public health effort. Dave had expressed similar opinions.

"And then can you get him to wear a mask?" Tara asked. "And can you also get him to wear a mask when he goes and golfs with his buddies? And then when he goes into the clubhouse and has drinks afterward? Because in that case, yeah, that's probably good. But if people see him giving one message and then living by another set of rules . . . ," she trailed off.

I knew she was right. Just like President Trump undermined public health messaging at the national level, some vocal business leaders who held a great deal of power may have been undermining public health messaging at the local level. In a few days the board of supervisors were planning to meet on the upper level of Parks Marina with business leaders and state legislators, including local Republican representative John Wills, to fundraise for the Republican party.[9] These business leaders held all the power to determine when and where public health recommendations would be enforced because there was such a weak federal and state response.

Others have written about the need for local leaders to collaborate with public health leaders, suggesting, "The consequences of an incoherent response, coupled with the impacts of impaired legitimacy, have grave implications: they have allowed an already serious threat to dig in deeper, leading to a longer crisis and thousands more deaths that might otherwise be the case."[10] The greatest promise, they suggest, is civic partners, health professionals, public health departments, and politicians working together.

Tara went on, "You do know people appreciate Zach though, right? Like I know he feels like he's probably banging his head against the wall. But there's so many people who appreciate what he's doing." I was beginning to wonder if it was worth the Herculean effort the public health team was devoting to their response when the hospital and county public health department had such limited authority, and the messaging was seemingly being undermined by local leaders.

The local business leaders' undermining of the public health effort reminded me of *Stories in the Time of Cholera*, a book about cholera in Venezuela by anthropologists Charles Briggs and Clara Mantini-Briggs. They found that political leaders similarly put the onus of responsibility on the community afflicted by cholera and blamed local people for the outbreak, considering them unsanitary. In doing so, local leaders often used racial profiling. Briggs and Mantini-Briggs wrote, "citizens were exhorted to assume personal responsibility for cholera control at the same time that they were expected to recognize that they were participating in a collective effort—and to recognize the authority of MSAS [the ministry of health] to direct it. An outbreak of cholera should bring people together, not give rise to partisan politics and attacks on the government and its institutions."[11] During the coronavirus outbreak in the United States, health authorities held limited power to implement public health measures when the federal and state governments failed to act. But similar to the cholera outbreak in Venezuela two decades before, the onus of personal responsibility deflected blame from a lack of political leadership to local people who navigated competing personal and social expectations. Although structural racism played a role in the Venezuelan case, a blur of white exceptionalism was happening in Okoboji.

Tara reflected, "And when it comes down to personal responsibility, we can all do everything right most of the time. But we make that one exception and that maybe gets us sick. Well, then somebody else makes that one exception around them and that gets them sick. So even if people are trying to do mostly what's right, we're not all encouraging each other to do the same thing."

Language around right and wrong, real and imagined, was complicated, especially when America's federal policy was, as stated by the White House Coronavirus Task Force coordinator Dr. Deborah Birx, that people would "Do the right thing." She continued, "Right now, we gain freedom through wearing our masks and socially distancing."[12] Doing the right thing, in this message, was clearly pointed toward conservatives who were against government involvement in their lives. But the problem is not that people did not want to do the right thing. Instead, residents looked to leaders, such as Trump, Reynolds, local mayors and political leaders, and business owners, whose actions seemed to indicate that they believed coronavirus mitigations impeded personal freedom.[13] Lina Tucker Reinders of the Iowa Public Health Association said, "When our strategies are not consistent with CDC evidence, when we are not adhering to even the advice of the White House task force, it raises questions in people's minds on the seriousness of the pandemic and the validity of the mitigation strategies." She continued, "People don't necessarily know what the right thing to do is."[14]

CHAPTER 6

SHAME

NOT EVERYONE IN the business community acted this way.

"You know Maxwell's did a fabulous job. They had a suspected case and they immediately shut down for two weeks," my classmate Lisa told me. Lisa is an old friend who describes herself as very conservative, religious, a Fox News devotee, and a successful businesswoman. She completely flipped the conservative stereotype about what she might think about coronavirus on its head. Lisa said, "I'm a prepper, like a nervous-Nellie prepper. So, I heard about coronavirus back in February when it really was not an issue here at all. People thought I was a little crazy. I went out and I pre-bought masks when I heard about it. I was like, when it actually started here, I was completely prepared. Like I had everything already ready."

I laughed and said, "Like other people got toilet paper, you got your masks?"

Many business owners I spoke to were concerned about public health guidelines. But I don't think my sample was necessarily representative of the business community at large; hundreds of people ignored my emails, texts, Facebook messages, and calls in the form of silence, or a kind reply stating that they couldn't step away from the hustle for even a quick chat. Others simply said, "I'm not interested!" or pointed to the political environment as being too hot to talk. Slow uptake is common in this type of ethnography, where you talk to as many people as you can through snowballing. This means that you reach out to one person who puts you in touch with another person. You have to shrug when someone ignores you and keep contacting people until you find enough who will talk to you. But it's safe to say that many of the people who were not interested in following public health guidelines were also not interested in participating in a research study about COVID-19.

For this research study, I analyzed the statements of ninety-nine people, collected from eighty-six in-depth interviews and thirteen testimonials in public forums. Twenty-eight of these people owned their own businesses. The rest worked in the hospital, schools, politics, nonprofits, and health centers. Some described multiple jobs or shift work at large national or regional stores, restaurants, cafés, gift shops, grocers, or manufacturing plants. Most people I spoke to were middle or upper middle class. About 12 percent described low wages, and one quarter earned very high wages. Three in four people I spoke to had completed college or more schooling. The rest had finished some college, technical school, or high school.

Among those formally in the research study, seven people said they were politically independent, mentioning that their minds were not made up about the 2020 election. Forty-one people identified as Republican, and five more said they were moderate Republicans. While some of these people were unwavering Trump supporters, others felt conflicted—between a rock and a hard place—because the politics around coronavirus conflicted with their preferred political identity. The three Libertarians were similarly conflicted about the election. Forty people reported they were Democrats. One young person said she was unsure about politics. I describe this demographic makeup here because, although the community slants far to the right, my sample was somewhat balanced politically.

DO YOU CARE ABOUT ME?

I spoke with a number of business owners who were taking COVID-19 precautions very seriously, and they described in detail how science and CDC guidelines influenced their decisions. None of these businesses completely shut down. Instead, nearly every business owned by the people I spoke to that was serving the public was open by appointment only or regulating how many people could enter their store at once. For example, Yoga Okoboji, my favorite local yoga studio, offered only online or outside classes for many weeks; later they opened with limited capacity indoors. Down the road, the Barn Swallow, an eclectic local gift shop, required masks and provided them free of charge at the door. Most contractors and realtors met with clients outside, on the phone, or by appointment in an airy meeting room. Many of these business owners were concerned with their patrons feeling safe.

Some of these business owners were beyond frustrated by what they saw other business owners and community members doing throughout the pandemic. For example, I spoke with a business owner, who I will call Merin, who was deeply rattled by the community's resistance to masking. Merin was a "blueberry in a can of tomato soup." I heard this expression from an old friend who used it to describe her own cultural deviance as a Democrat in Dickinson County. There could not be a better Iowan expression. It made me laugh so hard my belly hurt.

I sat with Merin at a small table in the back of her shop. We both wore masks, and she wore a face shield and gloves. We spoke for about an hour. There were long pauses between topics, which felt so natural I wanted to stay there all day. Merin was thoughtful and tender, communicating how deeply unsettling it had been for her to observe the community shift away from caring for each other. For her, the anti-mask stance was moral as opposed to political.

When I asked what people can do to prevent coronavirus, Merin provided the most lucid moral argument I had heard. "Well, I think of course, masks. Unfortunately, it's a statement in itself. It's a statement to wear a mask to protect or assist with someone else's well-being. And to choose not to do that is much more of a statement about who you are than what your political opinions align with. So, to me, it's more of a character type of, I guess that's a personal opinion, because if you're unwilling to care for someone else's well-being, then I take offense to that. Because that's what it is. You're helping others, for other community persons. You're not protecting you. But other people around you."

I shared how surprising it was to arrive to the Lakes and see so few people wearing masks. "From your perspective and from your observations," I asked, "what are you feeling and what do you think is behind this?"

"Well, honestly it has changed my perspective even driving down the road now," Merin explained, "because I'm viewing humans differently as to how they are caring about other people. And so, if they have so little disregard for other people, how are they going to be driving the fastest vehicle, you know? I have all of these other mind-boggling perspectives on human nature that have stemmed from this. That I feel we have strayed so far from the general moral of what it is to be human, and what it is to live in a community to take care of one another."

I thought back to Dutch philosopher Annemarie Mol's critique of logics of choice in this moment.[1] In what ways were people making these choices: To mask or not to mask? To drive fast or drive slow? What did choice mean anyway? Mol argues that instead of a logic of choice, we should think about these circumstances as involving a logic of care. Situating within a logic of care imbues the decision with greater meaning that has a backstory and front story, a history and present. This means that decisions around risk for an individual or community must involve aspects of *caring* for people—truly seeing their needs, complexity, and feelings. Caring is something that grows out of mutual knowledge and engagement in promoting good health and whole lives (as opposed to decisions chosen moment to moment without a history or community of people). Although Mol speaks about caring within clinical contexts, there is relevance to community contexts where logics of care determine people's actions, especially when those actions have serious implications for others. In this way, people were not making a choice to mask or not: they were demonstrating their motivation to care (or not) for others.

"And there is a lack of humanity in it," Merin stated with certainty in reference to people avoiding masks.

"Why do you think it is happening? That is definitely really different than other places in the country," I responded. "What do you think is behind it?"

"I think power," Merin said, shifting in her seat and resting her chin on her hand. "And it is having that sense of power to make that decision. And if you are a person that needs that sense of power then you don't have that power somewhere else in your life."

"That is really smart," I replied, scribbling a note about how people who have lost power and feel disenfranchised often exercise it in different ways. Rejecting masks, as she so clearly pointed out, was a way to exert power when someone felt powerless. As Francis Fukuyama explained in his book *Identity*, "while the economic inequalities arising from the last fifty or so years of globalization are a major factor explaining contemporary politics, economic grievances become much more acute when they are attached to feelings of indignity and disrespect."[2] In this way, people who resist masks but repeatedly miss work because they become sick or are exposed to coronavirus (and possibly become financially crippled) exemplify the politics of resentment in American society that enabled the rise of Donald Trump.

"At least what I'm seeing here, I don't like to generalize different groups. But I think, at least what I witness in the store, there is a lot of masculine energy in people who don't like to wear masks. So, it is a lack of grounding, and lack of connection with who they are. There is just something they can utilize to feel powerful."

I paused, meditating on her masculine energy trope—the forceful and assertive yang to the feminine and nurturing yin. Could acts of mask-defiance illuminate an outward expression of power and control over an unfamiliar threat? I found her comment fascinating and mulled over the possibility that perhaps rejecting masks reflected a deeper patriarchal thread in Okoboji. In northwest Iowa, where they are largely expected to be breadwinners, men hold on tight to traditional gender roles. It may be that men feel their identities threatened by financial loss to the pandemic. Could these idealized norms play out in shaming mask-wearers and throwing their energy into the economy? This reminded me about Jonathan Metzl's comment that "according to evolutionary biology, these men responded in predictable ways [when their masculinity felt threatened]—by smoking, fighting, drinking, pumping iron, driving too fast, or other modes of chest-beating that restored a sensation of order but also increased their blood pressures and shortened their collective life spans."[3] Is their rejection of masks perceived—maybe not outrightly but deep down—as an investment in their communities?

A few days later, Merin closed down her shop and offered customers the option to pick up items at the front door exclusively for the rest of the summer.

THE SHAME OF SHUTTING DOWN

Lisa was the first person I spoke to who emphasized how much she appreciated Zach's efforts. "There are so many rumors now that we've got this terrible outbreak. There are so many bad things on Facebook and people are sharing all this information. And I don't even know how he is finding the time. But he is literally going on these news pages on Facebook and correcting people and stopping fearmongering. I'm just so impressed with him."

It was comments like these that made me realize that dispelling myths and rumors was the most powerful arsenal Zach had for the public health effort. Facebook was a powerful tool in spreading rumor and creating disbelief within the community. Throughout the summer, people would talk about Facebook indirectly in conversation. "They said . . ." "Someone posted an article . . ." These indirect comments illustrated how commonly people engaged on Facebook and how the "imagined audience" among people in the Iowa Great Lakes was neighbors and friends, some close and others living far away who had some stake in the community.[4] This audience was often carefully culled; people would comment, "If I see something I don't like, I unfriend them," and "I spend so much time clearing up my newsfeed"—suggesting that they unfriend, block, or silence people who they disagree with. What happened in the

Okoboji Facebook community (and around the world) was an infodemic—where there was *too much* information, and many people found it difficult to parse fact from fiction.[5] Infodemics involve information about the epidemic that addressed risk, responsibility, and prevention, including some information that was true and a lot that was false.[6] Zach would often disappear with his phone when we were hanging out with the kids. My sister would pivot and say, "Where did Zach go?" Zach was literally breaking down myth and disbelief as it crept up on Facebook.

When I asked Lisa if things had changed since Memorial Day, she replied, "Oh, I definitely think that's changed. People are done, I mean they're over it. And the problem is that it couldn't come at a worse time, because now we have a serious problem here." I spoke with Lisa on June 17, two days after the first person from the Iowa Great Lakes had died from COVID-19. At the time, fifty-one Dickinson County residents had recovered from COVID-19, and 108 cases were active. The Iowa Department of Public Health had recorded 159 cases in total, with 135 of those cases occurring in the past two weeks.[7] People were starting to take notice, while others were losing interest in the public health effort altogether.

Lisa described the bus incident, seeming challenges with Parks Marina, and frustration with those businesses that acted like the virus would never touch them. But I wanted to know more about what she thought about Maxwell's Beach Café. I had just heard they shut their doors for the two weeks leading up to the Fourth of July weekend—when up to half a million people come to Okoboji and more than one thousand customers walk through their doors every day.

Maxwell's Beach Café is the place you go for your birthday, or to dress up and celebrate something special in the fancy dining room with deep booths, cloth napkins, and a wide bar; you can also sit on the outdoor patio and have a smaller menu. But the place is much more expensive compared to most restaurants in town. Like many longstanding businesses in Okoboji, it has become an institution. The longtime owners of the Café ran it for three decades, selling it a couple years ago to an old family friend of mine, Steven, and his wife, Leah. Leah was a social worker who threw everything into their new restaurant after they sank their money into it. The restaurant involves months of hard work with a long winter respite. This is a common lifestyle pattern among restaurant owners in Okoboji: spending the winter in Florida.

Steven and Leah hedged their bets and closed down the restaurant before the Fourth of July swarm after two employees tested positive for coronavirus. Steven conveyed in the *Dickinson County News*, "This is my decision for my restaurant for now. And it could be the completely wrong decision—I mean, if someone knows the answers to all this COVID stuff, they should step up and come forward." He also said, "You have to have money to survive but, at the same time, there has to be some kind of balance. I'm not going to take the risk of getting a staff member sick or one of our great guests sick for some extra money."[8]

Lisa said, "These really big establishments, they don't have a choice to close down. Then, you've got a nice little business, like Maxwell's, and they made the right decision. But you can't believe the community backlash they got."

I reached out to Steven to ask about the backlash. But he was too busy, or overwhelmed with the politics perhaps, to respond. I spoke to a close friend of theirs who said, "I feel like it's probably some of that Okoboji sentiment [that has made it so difficult] because nobody else is shutting down. They think that Maxwell's, because they did shut down, must have this huge problem." And by problem, she meant a huge outbreak. "When in reality, as far as I know, as of now, only four employees have tested positive and others have come back negative. I know one of the reasons, you know, Leah was really concerned about is, if you think about how Maxwell's works, they hire families. So, it might be that there's . . . ," she paused. "For example, I have a friend whose kids work there and she has twin daughters who are twenty-one and her eighteen-year-old son works as a bus boy. They all live in the family condo. They're from Omaha. So if one of those kids test positive, then the other two have to quarantine as well. And I think [Steven and Leah] are really worried about how they're going to staff the restaurant if they have an outbreak. And second of all, they have really been concerned about COVID from the get-go."

But there were major social consequences for Maxwell's decision to shut down. Lisa continued, "Yes, because people were saying to them, well you know you are insinuating that you know others in the community should follow suit with you. And that was not the case at all. I mean, the fact that he had to go on social media and explain himself."

"Oh, did he? I didn't see that, interesting."

"As a business owner, I—and I think differently than a lot of people 'cause I think from a business owner point of view—I didn't like that. It just didn't sit well with me that he had to go and explain his decision for making the right decision for his employees, for the community. You know, he certainly—I mean I reread that post three or four times—there was nothing in there to believe that he was insinuating that others should follow suit."

I asked why people got so mad about them shutting down. Lisa explained that it was much more complicated than it appeared. "We're just still small at the end of the day. But my personal opinion is they felt guilty. I mean, [the other restaurant owners] probably knew that it was the right thing to do and they knew financially they couldn't make that decision [to shut down for two weeks]. So, you know, I usually find that when people feel guilty, that emotion usually comes out as anger. A little bit of resentment."

I realized that Lisa was emphasizing that other businesses resented Steven and Leah for shutting down for two weeks because they felt shame that they would not or could not make the same decision. Their anger was directed at the fact that Maxwell's decided to do what many locals expected restaurants to do when they had multiple coronavirus cases: close down.

"You're talking about his Facebook post?" I read it closely as soon as we hung up the phone.

UPDATE: On Thursday, Dickinson County Board of Health and Lakes Regional Healthcare reported that 90 cases have been reported in Dickinson County, and the numbers in this area will continue to rise. The Lakes Area now ranks among the national hot spots for COVID-19 on a per capita basis. In other words, the virus is in our community, it is spreading, and our efforts to social distance remain as important now as ever.

We love Maxwell's because it is a place to come together, enjoy a meal, and spend time in good company. However, COVID challenges our ability to do so safely. Because we love our staff and patrons that make the magic happen, we have made the difficult decision to close for two weeks starting Monday, June 15th, to protect our community. We hope to participate in slowing the spread now so we can come together again, in love, come July.

We will miss the bustle while we are apart. If you feel called, please visit us in the coming days, in masks or for take-out, to help us avoid food waste when we close on Monday. We appreciate all the support you have given and continue to give us as we navigate this pandemic together.

We will welcome you back on Monday, June 29th, with—metaphorical—open arms. #dotherightthing #weloveourcommunity[9]

To me, this was an example of how someone might "do the right thing." I don't know the owners well, but I wondered if Leah's background in social work, a discipline devoted to protecting the community, influenced their decision to close down for two weeks. Their close friend told me that whenever negative messages were posted, "Leah's gotten them off right away." That made sense because when I scrolled through the thread, I could barely find anything negative about their decisions at all. This was because Leah had to carefully wipe away the smears to protect their business. Maxwell's, and the 100 days of summer, was their lifeblood.

"It was just a post," Lisa continued. "But the problem is that—you know, we're a small town. You remember what it's like, I mean," she paused. "That went viral, you know? I mean, that quick. Everybody was sharing the post and everybody, you know, everybody was texting a screenshot and texting it to everybody. Nothing is secret here."

SHAMING

I heard that some restaurants made a pact never to close down, even with active cases. They made this pact after Maxwell's shut down; they thought Maxwell's transparency was bad for business in the Iowa Great Lakes. When Maxwell's opened up, staff were in masks. The tables were spread far apart. The upscale restaurant was not taking any chances.

A coworker and friend of the owner of Maxwell's, Tom, said that when he asked Steven, "Might there be positive side effects here, good PR?," Steven told him, "I hope so."

Tom went on to explain, "But oddly he said, and I don't want to name names, but some very regular customers called him right after he closed down and they said, 'We are demanding to know why you closed! Are you giving into this fake concern?' And then there were some that were calling in saying, 'What is the real number of employees that are positive?' They were like, 'You would never have shut down unless it was half of you!' And Steve was like, 'It was just two and we want to make sure that it is not more.'"

In many ways, this direct confrontation was an implicit form of shaming. Shame is a powerful social tool. As a feeling of humiliation or distress caused by a perception of foolishness or wrongdoing, shame shapes how people think about engaging with others. Shaming is not always visible; but masks are. People wielded shame about masking and unmasking throughout the summer around the country, causing the choices people make about whether or not to put on masks when they leave their homes to be calculated and in many cases linked to fear that they may be judged.[10] Shaming can also be subtler, such as the tilt of a head, the scooting away of a chair, a laugh, or a stern look of disappointment.

The wealthy patrons who admonished Maxwell's for shutting down illuminated how many people wanted their bubble to stay intact, even if they largely stayed out of view to the public eye. I said, "So, loyal customers called him and attacked him?"

"I think he navigated it quite well. I don't know how well you know Steve, but he is like a happy, calm, friendly guy. I think it has been pretty easy for him to kind of say, and kind of say it with a smile, that 'we just want to be careful and we can afford to do so. I think it is in the best interest for you as our customers and our employees and our staff that we really care about.' So I think it was okay in the end, but I was fascinated to hear that, two things were going to happen, I would have thought, one, they would be commended and, two, I really thought that a few other places would follow suit."

"And no one did."

"No one followed suit," Tom confirmed. "Other restaurants shamed Maxwell's for closing down."

"Shamed them?" I asked to clarify. I started to wonder how much of this shaming was political and how much of it was related to financial survival. I concluded that it was definitely both.

"Yes. They are telling you that it's not dangerous to eat out. It's dangerous to eat out in restaurants that closed because that's where the cases are."

I thought this was an astute observation because shaming is a cultural script that serves at least two important purposes. First, it makes people feel part of something bigger by ascribing to a "script" or rules within a group. Second, shaming can coerce others to conform to a particular set of beliefs, such as masking (conveying support for left-leaning politics) or unmasking (supporting right-leaning politics).[11] In many ways, this is how in-group, out-group pressures played out throughout the summer. This is how shame was used among restaurants during the summer when coronavirus ran through the waitstaff around town: after Maxwell's was shamed, others hid positive COVID-19 cases among their employees to avoid any sort of public shame.

"Okay, give me an example," I asked Tom.

"The Lounge at the Inn, for example. From being in high school with the lady who runs it and following her on social media, I know that she was one of the ridiculers" of Maxwell's, Tom explained. The Lounge was another fancy restaurant at the Lake that had growing numbers of elite clientele. It was widely known around town that the owners of The Lounge at the Inn advocated for herd immunity and, at least in June, put only limited public health measures in place. "She [the owner] was voicing that it was great to open public places because, if there is any concern, it builds natural immunities and also [reduces] the need for a vaccine, which [she says] is going to cause autism. So, that is kind of . . . ," Tom trailed off, indicating that he disagreed with the restaurant owner's alleged conspiracy theories.[12]

Another local Democratic politician explained this in greater detail a couple weeks later. "I think that the lack of leadership [in making coronavirus policy] from the governor's mansion and especially our state rep here, John Wills, really puts a lot of pressure on businesses to take the lead. Like the Jensens down at Maxwell's. You know, closing on their own during the high season, to try and turn the tide on this thing. You know it's unfortunate that they had to be the ones to take the lead there. Meanwhile, Representative Wills has been using this mask issue and framed it from very early on the mask issue as an attack on our liberties and freedom. And framed the shutdown of the area as an attack on our liberties and freedom."[13]

In mid-June, closing down a restaurant because there were positive cases among the staff appeared anything but extraordinary. I could not understand then why it would be unusual for a busy restaurant to close down when two staff members had a contagious disease that could harm customers. Was the controversy about shutting down an attack on left-leaning politics? The business owners in this case were not openly political. Yet, in the end, their actions were extraordinary. No other restaurant in the Iowa Great Lakes closed down in those early months because there was no incentive to. In contrast, if they did consider shutting down, the example made out of Maxwell's showed that they had a lot to lose.

TRADE-OFFS

When I was scrolling through local friends' Facebook pages, I saw someone repost a message from a server in a restaurant. She posted, "Anyone who is shocked restaurants are hiding COVID positive employees and ignoring public health guidelines has never worked at a restaurant. If you have dined out with any regularity in your life, you've 100% been waited on by a feverish server who's been throwing up in the back because they would be fired and starve if they stayed home because no one wanted their shift."

I stopped scrolling, thinking about what this post meant and how deeply broken our society has become. It reveals how risk is overshadowed by the need for money, or what medical geographers Matthew Sparke and Dimitar Anguelov describe as "a ghoulish cost-benefit calculus of trade-offs [. . .] in which the economic benefits of opening shops or factories or whole cities and states is either implicitly or explicitly weighted against the costs of new deaths."[14]

The server's post underscores the stress of work in America, and how American culture and capitalism provide very little leeway to workers who face sickness, exhaustion, or fear. This was a common feeling among workers in Okoboji during the summer of 2020. I spoke to a number of employees of other restaurants about whether Maxwell's made a good choice in shutting down.

A young bartender said, "I thought that it was smart for them to shut down. I remember talking with my co-workers, and I was like, isn't that nice that they shut down for two weeks?" The bartender went on to describe their place of work, "And I'm like Captain's [Getaway] would never do that. Like our bosses are anti-social distancing, anti-masks, anti-everything." She seemed matter-of-fact, and continued, "And I get it because they are looking out for the business. But also, you have to look out for your employees sometimes."

The bartender went on to describe how the bar alleg-edly hid cases. "I remember I got mad that one of our waitresses tested positive, but that [the owner] didn't tell any of us, which I know that might have been a violation of her privacy." I scratched my head and thought, *where were the contact tracers?* She went on, "But I remember I was on the boat with one of my good friends and she was like, 'I heard so and so from Captain's has tested positive!' And I was like, 'I didn't know that.' I worked with her the other day and so a lot of us at Captain's had the antibody for it or had tested positive. But it was never put in like the group message, like 'hey guys, so and so has it, just like be careful.' There was never anything like that," she grimaced. "I think it was good for Maxwell's to do that but Captain's would never do that."

I decided to speak to Julie Mau, the owner of the big boat retailer Mau Marine and popular restaurant the Oko-boji Store. She owns these businesses with her sister. They bought the marina from their father, who bought it from Wilson Boat Works—one of the first in the Iowa Great Lakes. For ninety years, three generations of Wilsons had provided spaces for visitors and residents to pick up supplies and socialize. People rode in on horse-drawn carriages, steamships, and wooden boats. The Wilsons also operated a swing bridge.[15] I remember the store the Wilsons ran, however, as a Kentucky Fried Chicken. It wasn't until 2015 that the Mau sisters bought it back and transformed it into the iconic Okoboji Store.

The Okoboji Store is both a bar and a restaurant with layered decks. You can travel there by boat, car, or bike, and look out over the water. The Okoboji Store is located on the strait between East and West Lakes, and enmeshed with Mau Marine. It has affordable upscale food, a great bar, and a huge outdoor patio with a big playground for the kids to run and play while their parents relax. There is often live music, which always draws my kids in to dance, clap, and sing just as we are heading home to put them to bed. It is one of the places Lisa described in her description of the local economy: "It could be on any street in Minneapolis, you know? Or in Orlando, Florida! I just feel like there are so many people, something special—community members here that come with these amazing visions that bring places like that."

During the summer of 2020, the Mau sisters implemented strict coronavirus protocols—masking, social distancing, and periodic closures for cleaning. Lisa described the Okoboji Store as "doing the best job in the Lakes of COVID sanitation and, you know, everything else." There were outbreaks there, and rumors about positive cases. But it was also visible that they were trying to implement public health measures when few others did. They said they were following the CDC guidelines as well as those from the Iowa Restaurant Association. Tables were visibly spaced farther apart and there were fewer tables than in years past. The waiters wore masks and there was hand sanitizer everywhere. Few patrons wore masks. But the Maus did not think that they even could or should enforce masking among customers. Masking was perceived by many business owners as a problem of personal responsibility that business owners could not control without a mandate from a higher-level official.

By the end of June, the Maus had also dealt with two of the wait staff who had positive coronavirus tests. But they never closed down. Instead, Julie had developed an in-depth contact tracing system for her staff. She created a spreadsheet and had a restaurant manager closely track it. She recorded if a staff member was exposed, by whom, how, and where.

I was impressed to hear the lengths to which the Mau sisters went to design their system of tracking cases; if someone tested positive then they would trace cases among their staff. In many ways, their internal system rivaled the hospital's.

It was through this highly organized system that Julie figured out her staff was getting exposed to coronavirus at Millers Bay. She tracked a category called "house party" with a category called "Millers Bay," which came up over and over. She said it was so repetitive by mid-June that she felt compelled to call the public health department.

I spoke with Julie and others about the planning and techniques she put into tracking her staff and following the cases. Although she was not supportive of local or state government legislating her business, she was clearly taking the idea of "personal responsibility" seriously.

I spoke with Julie for nearly ninety minutes at the long table in the second-story conference room at Mau Marine's administrative building. I was there with my aunt Abby, and we all wore masks. The fresh lake breezes flipped through the open windows. We then spent another thirty minutes walking around the vast campus to see how she had adjusted business-as-usual to keep her staff and customers safe.

A week after we met with Julie, a close family friend texted me, "Julie Mau has coronavirus! You need to get tested." My cousin had dragged her family out of quarantine in LA and was driving, camp site to camp site, to visit Okoboji for the Independence Day weekend, arriving the next day. They got tested in LA, at stops along the way, and were planning to get tested again in Dickinson County. When Abby and I heard the rumor, my cousins were furious with me. How could I have put their mother at risk? I was frustrated, too. We got tested, and waited anxiously for the result. My dad spoke to Julie the next day, and found out she had been neither exposed nor positive. But the local rumor mill, which runs rapidly through a small town, was on fire.

CHAPTER 7
PIN FEATHERS

EVERY YEAR MY sister processes her first batch of one hundred chickens the day before the family descends on Okoboji for the Independence Day weekend. Kate is an organic farmer, raising perennial pasture with native grasses and pastured pigs and poultry. My kids usually fight over who gets to go with Auntie to move the chickens around the small eighteen-acre farm throughout the summer. She has ten pigs who live on rotated pasture and processes three batches of one hundred chickens per summer. They sell like hotcakes.

Usually, I pluck pin feathers on processing day—the easiest job. My dad puts a scalpel to the neck of the chickens and drains the blood. Zach scalds them and removes the feathers; Adam also scalds chickens and talks with Zach a mile a minute. My mother, sister, old family friends, and whoever else is on hand, including our kids, gut the birds and collect the hearts and livers into little bags. Then they throw the chickens into a chiller tank to cool. I pluck any remaining pin feathers with Abby once the birds are good and cold. The pin feathers don't require a lot of skill so

Abby and I talk for hours with whoever is helping for the day. It's the social table.

This year we spent a couple hours chatting up Sarah, a friend who dropped by to help on the farm. Sarah was one of the first COVID skeptics I met and talked with at length, in part because I had her cornered between chicken guts and pin feathers. I asked to record our conversation but Sarah declined, as many skeptics did. I was surprised by her beliefs because Sarah's husband was a local physician (who I will call Ted). Both of them were very outspoken about their resistance to public health interventions like masks for COVID-19. There were still around fifty new cases per week when we spoke, although the numbers had dropped some since the summer peak of cases in mid-June. It was in that moment plucking chickens when Abby and I began to understand why people believed coronavirus was a hoax and how some of the medical community may have been actively undermining the public health effort by telling people in the community that coronavirus was no longer a threat. This conflation of risk and reality was personal to me, and my family, with Zach entangled in the local response.

Learning why some people did not believe coronavirus was real or a risk to people in Okoboji was fascinating to me as a medical anthropologist. It reminded me of discussions with my classmates about magical thinking in my anthropological theory seminar with Professor Robert Launay at Northwestern University in graduate school. So often anthropologists discuss ideas about ritual, folk religion, or superstitions as things other people believed, in faraway places. But anthropologist Claude Lévi-Strauss argued that perhaps magical thinking was as common at home as it was elsewhere. He suggested that some people may actively use magical thinking to grapple for control over their environment.[1]

I probed her: Why do you think that? Where did that come from? Why is it a risk in other places, but not here? I was fascinated to focus on how folk theories were emerging in real time in my hometown.

But I wondered what damage local doctors like Ted might do. I spoke to many people who mentioned that a couple of local physicians conveyed mixed messages in contrast to those from public health leaders. I overheard people discuss the actions of these physicians—not wearing masks around town, telling people that coronavirus was over—in everyday talk.

I also received personal emails from concerned grandchildren (who I knew through my family's church or from childhood). They said Ted told their grandparents that they were not at risk for coronavirus; they emailed me asking if I could convince Zach to squeeze them in for a quick clinical visit. (Unfortunately, I did not have that kind of power.) They feared that this misplaced advice could cause real harm to their grandparents.

These messages increased throughout June. People often suggested to me that not all physicians agreed with Zach. Was coronavirus as bad as they say? Not here! There was more than one medical perspective on the pandemic.

The influence of these physicians grew in part because there were minimal consequences for their misgivings for nearly a year. The family physicians work for a Catholic healthcare system based in Sioux Falls, South Dakota, called Avera. Avera has slowly bought up small private clinics throughout the Midwest, creating different systems of care. Although there was oversight within the clinical space for medical deviance, much of the messaging of this particular physician occurred off-hours. Some of the harmful messaging went largely unchecked for months because the clinic itself was not governed by the local hospital and was somewhat disconnected from the Iowa Department of Public Health and the county supervisors' jurisdiction. Avera has little power to control what doctors say, and it takes a lot to fire or silence a physician, even when they are spewing untruths that may be harmful for community members. This is one example of how America's health system is fragmented and decentralized, making a unified health message difficult to maintain.

Even more, because so many physicians and nurses did follow the COVID-19 guidelines closely, and worked feverishly to support those sick in the community, this point emphasizes how important a unified policy is when one or two vocal dissenters can potentially cause public harm.

People started whispering about these conflicting messages. One health worker stated, "I read an article about Singapore early on and how their messages are coming from one source. And they posted the same message everywhere. It was—they got it texted to their phone, it went to an email, it was posted outside, like everybody had the same message for whatever period of time that was. And I don't think they had a hard time in Singapore and they knew like, they trusted their message. We have too many messages. And so nobody knows what to trust."

LOGIC OF CARE

But it was not only the two physicians that seem to have caused confusion about what COVID-19 was and how the community should respond. Many people's engagements with coronavirus were nuanced. For instance, a classmate who was a very public supporter of President Trump was also vocal about having a positive COVID-19 test and carefully quarantining with his family. He posted a photo of himself on Facebook with his wife and two children at home with the following message: "Living it up at our place we call home as we cannot leave and yes the rumor is true, My amazing wife and I have both tested positive for covid! Love your families!! #buildingourimmunesystems. #day7andcounting"[2] I was impressed by his openness about their diagnosis and taking the care to quarantine. Later he sent me a message saying, "I just wish people would not have so much fear," mentioning in the same note that he'd had COVID-19 twice.

Fear was central to so many people's coronavirus experiences. But it manifested in different ways, for different reasons. And fear was something I spoke about a great deal with people who made strategic decisions about when to mask, with whom they would interact, and what they would do.

Annemarie Mol argues that a logic of care "is not preoccupied with our will, and with what we may opt for, but concentrates on what we do."[3] One friend described this type of logic with regard to masking: although she did not perceive herself to be high-risk for moderate or severe COVID-19 and rarely wore a mask to protect herself, when she was around someone who was high risk, she put a mask on. She also described putting on a mask among those who were fearful, or who felt very strongly about others wearing a mask. She described very clearly adapting to the collective fear when it made sense to do so, even while caring differently for herself when she perceived it was comfortable and safe.

I spoke several times with a couple of friends who always made me think in a different way about things. We spoke in June and then again in late July. One friend explained to me, after putting in a great deal of thought: "I think probably some of your friends, I was thinking about this earlier today, you know I think people that are maybe in education or science or medical field right now, are just seeing things differently than the rest of us are. [. . .] Because what I'm seeing is, I don't even know anyone very close to me that has tested positive. I know of people. And of those people that I know most of them have recovered in a couple of days. So, I don't see a reason to be, you know, I personally don't have reasons to be fearful."

"And I do think that is something that is common here," I replied. "I mean five or six people have died now. But compared to DC, I have had lots of friends that have had it. I have a very close family friend that is in the hospital right now."

"I just feel that there is not enough logic going on," she replied. "There are the rules: they don't make sense. Six feet is such a stupid number. I think you know being out in the fresh air," she paused and shook her head. "I don't know how that got all tangled up with this. Why people wear a mask when you are out and about when you are away from people? I just feel like things have gotten messed up." I nodded as she spoke, because I found the shifting recommendations confusing myself, and I never wore a mask when I ran outside across the prairie or around the lake throughout the summer.[4] There was nobody around. Why should I?

My friend continued, "Maybe it is political. I don't know, I don't even follow politics." Many people in the wellness community said they didn't want to get entangled in politics. There was too much drama and they did not have the energy for it. Much of the focus within this community is on centering the self, looking inward before projecting outward. However, by saying that they are apolitical, they are actively taking a stand: ignoring politics is a political act in itself. Yet there was a widespread social contract to building peace of mind and supporting each other.

"But I feel that things have gotten messy and I'm just going to live my life," she explained. "Like I told you before, my friend, her dad died of COVID. He was the first one in Minnesota. And he was ninety-three, not that that was an excuse. He lived a great life, he wasn't sick. But you know, he was ninety-three. So he was in assisted living and however he got it there, he got it and he died within four days. And that is terrible, right? So, [my friend] masks all the way, stays away from people. She is a yoga teacher, studio owner. She is not going back to the studio. She doesn't plan on it. In fact, she sent her studio off with another teacher. So, I mean, I imagine if it impacted you in such a negative way, you would be fearful. But I feel logically if [my friend] looked at it, she would say my dad was ninety-three and he could have gotten pneumonia. He would have died, you know? So, let's be logical about this. Why are we going to stop living for fear?"

Fear was a contested emotion throughout the summer: some people were so fearful they would not leave their house, while others I spoke to were very clear that they did not fear coronavirus. A local therapist told me that there was very little care-seeking for fear associated with getting sick from COVID-19; some people sought care for anxiety and depression, and most preferred this care in person without masks. This contrasted acutely with my community of fellow academics and friends who work in public health. I constantly observed their texts, emails, Twitter, and Facebook feeds that conveyed the deep-seated anxiety, fear, and depression that was settling in across the country. In many ways, these friends were living in a constant state of fear, anxiety, and exhaustion. A reporter in the *New York Times* described "struggling with the emotional long-haul of the pandemic" as languishing, or "muddling through your days, looking at your life through a foggy windshield."[5]

The local therapist explained, "There is not a high level of fear, in my opinion, overall of COVID [in the Iowa Great Lakes]. There is just not. There are some, like I said, there is a high level of fear related to it [because of their personal risk or the risk of a loved one]. But overall, I'm not seeing that. I really thought that when I offered telehealth versus in office, that it would be a much higher percentage that would stay telehealth. I was shocked [when nobody chose telehealth]."

The therapist went on, "I hate to bring politics things into it, but I think it is more of a conservative thing. I think people here tend to—not all people, but a lot—tend to hold on to the belief they don't want government telling them what to do. And so to be told we are required to wear a mask doesn't feel good to a lot of people."

ENOUGH

A chiropractor I spoke to explained the divergence in views further. During the early months of the pandemic, she described how fear and anxiety around the virus wrapped around the community. However, since summer had set in, she described a calm that had settled upon the community.

"You know some people were really panicking, and you could feel, you could sense it. I just tried to tell them that stressing out about it actually weakens your immune system. You're actually doing yourself the opposite of good here, as far as trying to stay healthy in this time."

I followed up, "From a chiropractic perspective, what guidance do you give? What kind of dialogue do you have with people?"

"Well, most of it is just reassuring them that your body is an intelligent organism. It has the ability to fight these things if you give it what it needs. So, obviously you should be washing your hands. You should be staying home if you feel sick. I mean those are not new phenomena. Those are things you should be doing all the time. All year round." I smiled in agreement with her, thinking about how critical good hygiene was and how these new behaviors might become normalized, benefiting society as a whole. She went on to talk about things like handwashing and explained she was "trying to explain to people, you know, it's a virus, but it's just this family of viruses that has been around. This is not new, you know." Yet, by definition, an emergent infection like SARS-CoV-2 *was new*. It was zoonotic, meaning the virus had recently moved from animals to humans. There was so much we did not know.

I asked, "And how have you seen things change since things have opened up?"

The chiropractor continued, "I mean I think that hysteria has died down to some degree. I still have some people that are [worried] because they are immunocompromised, or they have someone at home who's immunocompromised. Things like that. For those people, it's still palpable when you talk to them. You can still feel it." The chiropractor went on to describe how this fear has shifted over the pandemic months, explaining the communal fear people felt at the beginning of the pandemic and the lingering fear felt mostly among those who were deemed high risk when summer came. This notion of who should fear and who should let things go was central to many conversations about risk, fear, and care.

"But I think some people have just kind of . . . ," she went on, ". . . you know, they've reached the point where they're just like, enough. Especially when Dickinson County was like hovering at eight cases for quite a while before

Memorial Day weekend. People then get to the point where they're like, is this even legitimate? You know, it's not increasing. I'm going about my life, you know. And . . . ," she paused, ". . . and it's hard to tell them like, no don't do that. But I think just encouraging them to continue to do those good practices is important."

"Do you think people are seeing it a different way or acting a different way?"

"I think some people have just reached the point where they're just like, I just don't care," she explained. I had been wondering what people didn't care about, and who.

The chiropractor went on to explain how people were thinking: "Like, 'I'm just gonna live my life and if I get it, I get it.' And I think for a lot of 'em, what I'm hearing is people say, some people are like, 'oh my gosh, the numbers are skyrocketing!' at least locally, here. And I'm like, 'yes, they are.' But also, we're testing now, more. I mean, like at the beginning of this when the testing was limited, there were people I know that said that they went in with mild symptoms that could potentially have been coronavirus, or could have just been a cold or something, and they were told, your symptoms aren't significant enough. Like we can't quote-unquote waste a test on you, essentially, for lack of a better term. And just go home and rest and recover at home. And if your symptoms increase, then let us know."

She shifted in her seat and continued to explain that she was somewhat science-skeptic. "So, I think now that the testing has increased and is more widely available, the numbers do look like they're going up, obviously. But, at the same time, people are like, well it could be on the downhill, actually. Like that's what you don't know. When you start testing more, obviously you're gonna get more positives, right? So I think some people have reached the point where they're like, 'well, is it really the curve they think it is, or are we actually coming down from it?' It just looks more dire right now because we're testing all these people. And, and I can't, I don't negate their rationale, you know? I'm like, yeah, it's a valid question. We'll never know that because we didn't test everyone all along since this started. You know, potentially back in December or January, or whatever. So . . ."

"There's some mistrust?" I interjected. I was hearing some common Republican talking points in this logic: the numbers don't mean anything; there is little one can trust.[6]

"Yeah, I think so. And, I guess I can't fault people for that," she responded. I nodded, wondering if her conversations with patients provoked some skepticism in the public health effort. "Like I mean," she said, "some people I think are willing to continue to stay home or wear a mask, you know, indefinitely until they're told, it's okay to go about your life." She tilted her head and said, "But there are some people that, I think they're just like, I'm not doing this anymore. Whether it's because it's affecting their job, their livelihood, or just their sanity. They can't just stay locked up. Or whatever, they're just over it." She stopped and laughed, tossing her head back. "But yeah, I guess I don't fault people either. It's all been a long time."

CHAPTER 8

FIREWORKS

ON JULY 4, 2020, the Lake was not as busy as expected. Usually, when you drive on Highway 71 from Wyman's Spudnutz donut shop, past the Okoboji Store, across the bridge from Okoboji into Arnolds Park, and toward the strip of bars on Broadway Street, you inch forward, with cars bumper to bumper. I remember years ago when my dad was two hours late to meet me for dinner in Chicago, slowed by rush-hour traffic on the Dan Ryan Expressway, he joked, "It was worse than Okoboji on the Fourth of July!" I could not stop laughing for the rest of the night. But the traffic was never bumper to bumper in 2020.

Zach woke up early and picked up donuts. Usually, we pre-order donuts at Spudnutz. But not this year. A week earlier Adam had snuck out of bed early to surprise the family with some sugary delights (our family indulges in these delicious morsels when the Okoboji heat gets thick). Locals and tourists alike get up before dawn to line up outside this donut shop; it's that good. But Adam did not realize he'd have to wait over an hour in a line outside the shop that weaved along the busy road to pick up a dozen

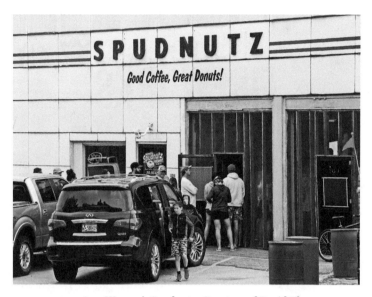

FIGURE 8.1. Wyman's Spudnutz. Courtesy of David Thoreson.

donuts. The kids were hangry when he got home and he was frustrated. "There were only a few people in line with a mask on," he said. "The guy at the counter thanked me for wearing a mask when I picked up the donuts. He told me that he was frustrated that so few people were." So when the Wyman's shut down their doors for the entire holiday weekend, regardless of the thousands of dollars they would lose, we were not that surprised. Zach picked up donuts at Hy-Vee, a regional grocer, instead.

I heard my sister shuffling around outside my basement window. I wasn't sure what she was doing, but it's usually some sneaky surprise for the family later in the day.

My mom and I met outside shortly after. I led a family yoga practice as we drank in the moments before the kids woke up while the lake was quiet. The sun was slowly inching up into the sky and the waves were lapping quietly, sounding like home.

After the sun was up and we finished our yoga, Adam walked over with my two perky kids. My cousin's five-year-old came shooting across the yard from Abby's house, shouting, "It's here! It's here!" He might have been talking about the holiday. But I'm pretty sure he meant the donuts.

We spent the morning in the lake. We ate sandwiches on the dock. It's the one moment in the year that I get together with my cousins, and we talk a mile a minute, while minding our rambunctious kids. We had all gone to extra lengths to quarantine, test, and gather.

By one o'clock, my sister started blowing her whistle. My mom and I had followed her to the yard a while before to set up the games. We set up a table, homemade megaphone, and dress-up clothes. Kate put eggs on reserve for the egg toss. She tied string to the trees for the donuts. Tables were spaced out for the beer. By the time everyone reached the yard, she was literally screaming into a big orange megaphone she had made from poster paper, "The Family Olympics are starting!" Kate was wearing a floppy hat with a British flag on it with a string you pull down to make two extended hands clap together. We made my British grandmother wear that hat for years; I still remember her giggle when she blew the whistle for each event.

The kids started everything off. The dress-up game. The three-legged race. The donut chomp, which was everyone's favorite: we literally have to eat a donut with no hands from a string strung between two old oak trees. Everyone was constantly giggling. (But there is always a little one in tears; this year, it was my kid, whose donut fell onto the ground.)

The adults took off next. We started with beer and ended, again, with donuts. For a minute we forgot that coronavirus existed at all. We ended the Family Olympics with the most competitive game: the cannonball jump. Each team chose two contestants to cannonball into the water. Usually my uncle Bert wins, but he didn't travel this year because of coronavirus. I think it's the first July Fourth celebration where I've been there but he hasn't. I've missed a couple when I was living abroad. The day slipped away so fast.

When the sun disappeared, my kids nearly passed out from an excess of sugar and fun. We threw on sweatshirts and met at the dock. We packed the family into the boat and nosed our way out into the Lake to see the fireworks.

We left early in case the lake was packed. But there were fewer boats than usual. I snuggled my four-year-old close, whose eyes were droopy because it was well past her bedtime. We turned on Campus Radio so we could hear the soundtrack to the fireworks.

The fireworks filled the sky at 10:07 p.m. I looked around and could see the barges packed with people. The beaches were lined with families, snuggled up in blankets looking out over Smith's Bay. Partiers drank at bars set up on large barges that floated on the water. People sat on their cars in parking lots, near bridges. Others sat on decks at restaurants or on private docks, public walkways, and sandy banks. The central body of the lake was congested with boats, with people blasting the Campus

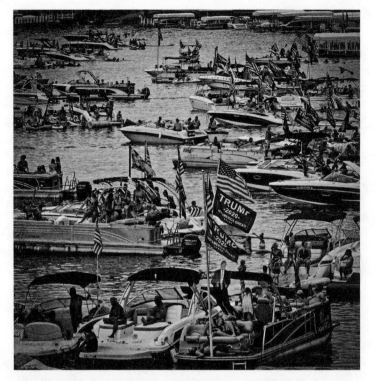

FIGURE 8.2. Trump flags pontoon. Courtesy of David Thoreson.

Radio program that accompanied the fireworks display. The display was paid for by the Iowa Great Lakes Chamber of Commerce.

Near the end of the fireworks, I laughed as my cousin Gerrit animated the increasingly patriotic songs. Campus Radio likes to pack a punch with the finale, playing "God Bless the U.S.A.," a "country anthem with enduring political power" in conservative politics.[1] I listened intently to the words as I hugged my daughter close. I thought about how differently people were thinking about notions of freedom as well as sacrifice amidst coronavirus. In many ways, they were in opposition in real life, although they were aligned in the patriotic verse.

In an interview with Don Gonyea, Lee Greenwood explained what inspired him to write "God Bless the U.S.A." He explained, "I wanted to put God first, because I'm a conservative Christian, and I wanted to make sure that God was honored in the song."[2] The song soon became an anthem for the Republican party, taking hold at the Republican National Convention that re-elected President Reagan and being played at the last four Republican inaugurations, including Trump's, advocating America First. It has become central to the Right's celebration of "liberty" and "freedom," and is expected to pull at your heart strings. Left-leaning reporter Arvin Temkar explained a few years ago that, despite liberals despising the song, he loves it: "The melody is an earworm, the swells are triumphant, and the emotion—though a bit syrupy—is authentic."[3]

What made me shake my head was the hypocrisy in this song amidst the coronavirus crisis. The mantra of individual freedom and personal responsibility was a powerful excuse for ignoring public health. "I'd thank my lucky stars / To be livin' here today / 'Cause the flag still stands for freedom / And they can't take that away."[4] But in this freedom a self-righteousness emerged that released people from responsibility for others. A moral disconnection was unleashed that rejected a notion of protecting the most vulnerable. "I won't forget the men who died, who gave that right to me."[5] But ideas of duty were ignored and people had died. In fact, someone died from coronavirus when the sun came up the following morning.[6]

NO SPARK

Iowa tourism data showed that there was still an influx of people, even if the roads weren't backed up. The data about arrivals, which were based on cell phone data of people who traveled at least fifty miles from home and spent more than two hours in Dickinson County (and who were over eighteen), tell an important story (although it excludes people with flip phones or no phones). The spring had normal numbers of visitors—in March (22,353 visitors) and April (26,567 visitors)—but there was a rapid increase in May (87,314 visitors) for Walleye Weekend and Memorial Day. There were again increases in June (105,290 visitors) and July (172,118 visitors). The Okoboji Tourism director Rebecca Peters told me that people assume the biggest influx of visitors is for the Fourth of July, but usually the second and third weeks in July are busier. From being there during that time, it did feel that the grocery stores and restaurants were constantly buzzing throughout July, but not packed like usual. Numbers dropped slightly in August (127,746 visitors), September (87,638 visitors), and October (47,550 visitors).[7] As raw numbers, these data appear enormous for a small county of seventeen thousand year-round residents, but they are slightly lower than usual.

Rebecca explained to Iowa Public Radio that there were fewer visitors during the summer because of coronavirus.

Many people booked last minute; she explained "they maybe decided on Thursday that they were going to visit that weekend" and "that allows them to see how our community's COVID numbers are doing to ensure that they're staying low and that the attractions that they want to visit will be open and following safety measures. But it also allows them to make sure that they themselves are healthy when they choose to come visit."[8]

We decided at the last minute to send our kids to day camp at Camp Foster YMCA in Spirit Lake. My sister and I attended the camp for years, first as day campers and then as overnight campers for a week at a time. Our kids have attended Camp Foster day camp for several summers. They love it because they get to swim, practice archery, learn new games, sing songs, get muddy, and eat candy. I was hesitant to put our kids in the day camp because of coronavirus, but as a board member of the camp, Zach had spent hours helping prepare social distancing plans. Everyone was outdoors and we hoped it would be safe.

What sealed the deal for me was watching a video of Laney, the social distancing officer, who composed a creative song for the kids to sing to make sure they were far enough apart. "Peanut butter, jelly," she said in a pink fairy costume while making wide swipes with her arms from her chest outward, "spread out! / Crackers and cheese!" she sang, "spread out please!" Then my favorite—"Oreo McFlurry / Spread out in a hurry!" She danced around with her arms open wide. "Make like a cow, and MOOve!"[9]

My kids were expert mask-wearers and I was confident they could follow the rules. From the beginning of the pandemic, we had explained to our kids the science and actions needed to prevent coronavirus transmission and why we had to wear masks to keep each other safe. If they wanted to do things around town (like get a Nutty Bar or go to the park), they would have to wear masks. It was amazing to see them slip into routines where they put on masks just as easily as they put on shoes.

But my intrepid boundary-testing youngest was a curious little kisser. She came home from camp on Thursday and told me, "Mommy, I kissed the new boy at camp. But don't worry because he was COVID-negative!" According to the little people who attended the camp, the little boy had a cough and could not attend camp until he showed a negative COVID-19 test (which I assume they did on Wednesday, and he told this to my daughter). She had a fever and cough by Saturday morning. I can't hold myself back from nuzzling, kissing, and snuggling my sick kids. So my sniffle and cough started a couple days later.

We went for COVID-19 tests the next Monday. The Test Iowa site in Spirit Lake was opened the last week in June and involved a drive-thru test at the Dickinson County Fairgrounds, where my nephew had proudly entered his first chicken in the county fair the summer before. It was incredibly easy to sign up for a test through the Test Iowa site. The directions about where it was located were clear. There were signs everywhere. When we drove up, a nurse scanned the bar code on our phones—one for each family member to be tested. Then they poked, tickled, and prodded our noses. I whined, but my four-year-old daughter giggled before she cried. We drove off.

Later they moved the testing site to a more central location near the YMCA, right outside the ice rink. It was similarly easy, although once I had to wait ten minutes because there was a line of cars. I heard other people complain about how long they waited to get their tests—but I never found that to be true. Others said their tests were mismatched with other people's tests. There was a false positive. A false negative. Someone had their results. But my assessment was that testing from the state was swift and seamless. Each time I tested, I received my negative results within thirty-six hours.

There were some discrepancies about what happened once the tests were sent off to the state and accounted for. But overall, the testing was reliable for the people who chose to get tested. My research suggested that most people who chose not to test either left town, thought it was a flu, or had no symptoms at all.

After the Independence Day weekend, cases did not shoot up like we expected they might.[10] A frequent argument was that most people working in restaurants and bars had had coronavirus in early June, so they reduced transmission over the holiday because they already had immunity. Another theory was that most people who were visibly out at bars, tying up in Millers Bay, or packed on party barges were tourists. When they left town, so did those cases of coronavirus. A local physician mentioned to me that his friends in Des Moines were frustrated by the influx of coronavirus cases from people who had visited the Lakes during the Fourth of July holiday.

It's hard to know how many people got sick from coronavirus over the Fourth of July weekend in the Iowa Great Lakes. It's impossible to measure. Even harder to contact trace.

But the reality is, the local population thought that, without the predicted spike, the worst was behind them.

CHAPTER 9

COMMUNITY TENSION

CORONAVIRUS INFECTIONS DID not spike over the Fourth of July. But community tension did.

I sat at a picnic table with a classmate and talked with her about how hard it was after she lost her job. I could see the stress wrinkled in her forehead, and her Midwestern suntan had bronzed her cheeks and shoulders. The wind whipped over the table between us. She had worked so hard to get that stable job—with benefits, reliable hours, and good pay. As the summer crept forward, she feared she would not be able to pay her bills. She was saving up to buy a house, but now she said that dream was gone. Coronavirus had taken away so much; people felt they had lost control over their lives.

Despite the relative wealth tourism brings the Iowa Great Lakes area, there are significant income disparities within the area that play out in everyday life. These tensions were starkest in the party district on Broadway Street where coronavirus reared its head and families balanced politics and safety during a time when they did not think the police would protect them.

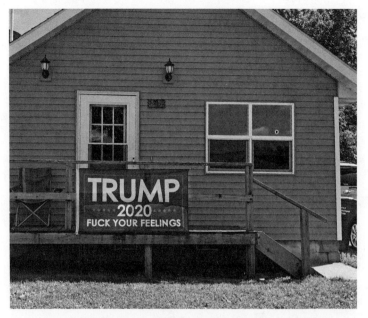

FIGURE 9.1. "Fuck your feelings" flag. Courtesy of David Thoreson.

I spoke with a middle-aged mom who I call Cheri, a mom who resided near "the strip," for two hours late one night after we had both tucked our kids into bed. She was one of many families who had a "Trump 2020" flag on the side of her house and I was looking forward to learning about why she felt so strongly about partisan politics. I expected a staunch Trump supporter who refuted the reality of coronavirus as a real threat to the community. But Cheri's experience provided nuance to political debate, and furthered my fear that business owners were acting against the safety of local families.

I connected with Cheri through a friend-of-a-friend who mentioned she was the one Trump supporter he knew who would talk to me. I called and texted her, but because she was managing so much without childcare or play dates for her four children, it took some time to connect. Eventually we found a quiet time to speak on the phone together. The call lasted for such a long time, with an out-of-state number, that her husband called me a few weeks later to see who his wife had been speaking with so long. He laughed, somewhat relieved, to hear that it was just the anthropologist she'd mentioned had been calling the house.

Cheri moved to Arnolds Park in her early twenties, living in the heart of the party district. She eventually settled down, married, and raised a family. When we spoke in July, Cheri was exhausted after months of struggling financially and caring for her four children. "Our year started out pretty normal," she said. "But then they let school out so I ended up quitting my job because I had to stay home with the kids. And daycare closed. And nobody wanted to watch anybody's kids because they were afraid they were gonna get sick." Cheri's situation was all too common for many women during the pandemic shutdowns.

Cheri's husband worked in a local factory, and the virus brought repeated financial problems with his work. Cheri explained that she felt shut-in in her home with her kids and struggled to figure out what to do with them. She said, "We couldn't take the kids to a store so our kids were really just locked in the house. We couldn't take them anywhere! We couldn't do that much. [My husband] was going to work all the time and then he ended up getting . . . ," the line went silent for a moment. "He didn't get infected but he was like . . . ," she paused again. "What's the word?"

"Exposed?" I asked.

"Yeah, exposed." Cheri went on to explain that he was on and off work several times throughout the spring and summer. They went weeks without any money coming in. Paying for food and rent continued to be a great concern for families throughout the pandemic in Iowa and around the world. Research during the 2020 pandemic year showed that eleven percent of adults in the US stated that their household sometimes or often did not have enough food to eat in the previous week. This was much higher than the usual three percent of families who didn't have enough to eat (and that was reflecting on the past twelve months). Most people identified "couldn't afford to buy more food" as the cause of going hungry (as opposed to barriers around collecting food like transportation or safety).[1] This was less common among white families than Black, Asian, and Latino families. Rent was especially hard to keep up with, and this was more common among adults with children like Cheri.[2]

Cheri continued to explain how financial uncertainty caused constant disruption: "The first two months he got paid two-thirds of a paycheck because of the family [leave]. And then the first time he was exposed at work they paid him his whole paycheck because it was work related. And then the second time he was exposed [outside of work], it was unpaid and he had to take two weeks off." She explained how frustrated she was with these two weeks of unpaid leave for quarantine because he had a negative test for COVID-19. I assumed the frustration was more about lost wages than the time spent at home.

"How'd you feel about that?" I asked.

"Uh, annoyed and angry," she huffed. "Because we didn't really get a say in the matter."

Cheri's comments made me think about what Lisa had said about friends and family members working in factories around town when they were forced to go back to work. She explained that many factories were "not observing any time off for quarantine" and "putting profit before employee health." She emphasized how this was happening in Dickinson County, and that it was even worse in the meat-packing plants in Storm Lake. I spoke to a technician at Polaris, a local company that makes motorcycles, snowmobiles, and ATVs, who said over the "past couple months they have done stuff to keep people at a distance. But some areas you can't." I asked if they wore masks on the factory line. The technician said, "Some people are required to wear a mask. But I just kind of float around so I don't wear a mask." A classmate who works as a security guard told me, "I refuse to live in fear. If something is going to happen, it is going to happen and there is not a damn thing I can do about it. I can go in wearing a mask but that doesn't mean that I still won't contract the damn thing." He went on, "So I wake up every day like it's a new day. And if I catch COVID, I hope I survive. But if I don't, I guess I'll just be another stat."

Americans were already struggling when coronavirus hit.[3] Cheri's story resembles those of many working families who struggled to make ends meet while facing increased risk of infection at work.[4] In her case, the threat was not only viral—it was also the reality of dwindling paychecks and lack of childcare. Droves of American women lost or left jobs, losing wages and security because of the pandemic.[5] These inequities were intensified among Black and Brown communities throughout America, including in the Midwest, who faced job loss amid a collective reckoning for racial, health, and economic justice.[6] Yet many white working-class families like Cheri's faced financial trouble that was far beyond that of their wealthier neighbors. Lisa indicated that the middle class "can work from home and they can afford to hire somebody to go get stuff for them." Lisa went on, "then you've got you know the upper class, who oddly enough . . . ," she sighed deeply. "I don't know, I feel like sometimes they feel a little invincible. A lot of those individuals I've seen are guilty of not wearing masks."

MASKS

Issues like masks accumulate larger symbolic or moral meanings in ways that rendered conversations about the effects of national and state coronavirus policies ever-more difficult.[7] Jonathan Metzl argued in his book *Dying of Whiteness: How the Politics of Racial Resentment Is Killing America's Heartland* that liberals are slow to realize how "Trump supporters were willing to put their own lives on the line in support of their political beliefs."[8] Focusing on contentious issues of gun control, health care, and school funding cuts, Metzl described how "frameworks of white racial resentment shaped debates about, and attitudes toward, various public policies and acts of legislation."[9] For instance, he provides the example of a woman who held on so tightly to her gun rights that she actually shot herself in the face while playing with her gun when her boyfriend drove off the road. She died by accidental suicide. In some ways, American practices of unmasking demonstrated a similar type of stubbornness. With the pandemic occurring amid the 2020 election, unmasking strongly aligned with President Trump's rhetoric of normalcy and downplaying of the severity of national outbreaks throughout the summer.[10]

Yet I noticed beliefs about masks were not clearly divided between right and left, wealthy and poor, religious and agnostic. Many people like Bethany, who was so frustrated that her kid was exposed to COVID-19 at work, were ardent supporters of President Trump while still advocating for masking and social distancing. Some conservatives were frontline workers at businesses that required masks and were relieved to have reliable masks to protect them. Others were in constant protest against being told to wear any mask at all. Some dangled their masks below their nose when their employer required them, in protest.

The most contested space in town, where maskers and unmaskers walked shoulder to shoulder, was Walmart. Walmart was the only place many people said they *would* mask. It was also the only place where there was national policy mandating that people *must* mask.

I found people across town grappled with Walmart after the corporation instated a mask mandate in mid-July.[11] Jay, the libertarian I spoke to who was conflicted about coronavirus but was certain there was a middle ground people could find, always put a mask on at Walmart. In contrast, a local politician told me he decisively avoided Walmart because he, as part of the GOP, would not be seen wearing a mask in public.

Walmart is located smack-dab in the middle of Dickinson County. It's at the intersection of Highway 9 and Highway 71, at a four-way stop that supposes low traffic and thoughtful onlookers. It's the type of intersection where my driver's education partner, Julayne, would grab the side of her seat and hold her breath (it took me several years to be confident behind the wheel). The parking lot is chock full throughout the year with mostly American sedans, minivans, SUVs, and trucks. People drive from around the county and neighboring towns to get supplies at Walmart: it's the biggest one-stop-shop for miles. In the summer, there are more luxury cars and the license plates reveal visitors from around the Midwest; you can also glimpse plates from California, Florida, and New York.

Walmart in Spirit Lake has become a local cornerstone not just of consumerism but also security. In many rural towns around the United States over the past several decades, the arrival of Walmart led to the shuttering of small businesses as it filled their market space with products and convenience. In high school, I mentioned at a classmate's house how Walmart was ruining the town and exploiting workers.[12] My classmate's mom sat down next to me and carefully explained how critical Walmart had become since so many people lost their farms.[13] When we started school in the eighties, thirty percent of my classmates lived on farms. Fifteen years later, less than five percent of my classmates lived and worked on farms. Watching the farming culture collapse around us had a huge impact on our generation. It was so visceral for my sister that she decided to devote her life to sustainable organic agriculture. But Walmart offered a secure job with health insurance linked to a national corporation for many families who left farming. It was accessible, reliable, and cheap for customers, as well as employees. You could pick up groceries and a new air conditioner in twenty minutes on your way home from a long shift.

Everyone mentioned Walmart in my interviews. It was a place where some people refused to go (on policy) but everyone would slip into (by necessity). I remember in mid-summer I took my eldest daughter and nephew to Walmart to spend some money they had earned from a (socially distanced, coronavirus-safe) lemonade stand. My eldest bought a kid's sewing machine and my nephew bought a Nerf Blaster. Walking through the store, we ran into people double masked with gloves and worried looks. The next beat we saw a man wearing a red flagship Make America Great Again hat with his mask around his chin.

What was striking about the anti-masking stance that so many people upheld was a simultaneous belief that if you were vulnerable, then you should stay home. Many people like Cheri—who often unmasked—balanced worry about someone they loved becoming infected and the perceived harm of masking. Cheri's child had a respiratory condition so she was concerned both with what might happen if her child developed COVID-19, and the conspiracy theory around CO_2 harming her daughter's lungs from wearing a mask all day. (Even though this conspiracy theory was widely debunked, it continued to spin.[14])

Yet masking was not a simple story. I spoke to a childhood friend who was up in arms with Dr. Fauci. Fauci had just gone on national television to encourage everyone to mask.[15] But it wasn't about Fauci encouraging people to mask—my friend wore masks all the time. He was enraged because in the spring Dr. Fauci had urged people to stop buying masks because of a limited supply for healthcare workers. My friend was a glassmaker but his wife worked in a hospital. When I asked Rebecca Katz about it, she explained a lack of personal protective equipment, or PPE, was in part due to Trump shutting down the pandemic preparedness program that fostered the strategic national stockpile of PPE. In many ways, my friend's struggles stemmed from these structural problems that impeded access to the PPE his wife required to do her job. Desperate to protect her, he drove to every Menards (a regional home improvement store) in the area to purchase masks— he cleared out shelves and packed them into the back of his truck.

TOURIST TRAP

"Unfortunately, in our area of Iowa, it always comes down to money over safety."

"Why do you think that's the case?" I asked Cheri.

"We live in a really tourist populated area, and if the state closed down like bars or restaurants or schools or things then the area would take a significant financial impact," she said. She emphasized that all the summer decisions to keep the economy thumping had been financial. Cheri explained, "If we just close things for a few weeks and let it ride out, I just don't think they could handle it. Like the financial impact they think would damage our area. But the people like us who live here all year long, we know that it wouldn't."

"That's so interesting," I responded. I was learning so much from her and thinking about the community in a completely different way. "I grew up in the area, I went to school with [our mutual friend], and now I live out east. I come back in the summers because my family lives here. What was so interesting is that we were in lockdown for a long time and then we got here and everything was open and we were like, 'This is just super weird.'"

"Isn't it?" Cheri said.

"Yeah. You think it's weird too?" I asked.

"I do. And we live here! But you know what would happen to the strip of Broadway if they shut them down. Like they would close. And they wouldn't be able to survive and the city of Okoboji and Arnolds Park is terrified. Arnolds Park being closed for one summer could've stopped so much of the spread of the disease around here. But because they needed that money and they needed that revenue, they opened it twice. Like they kept closing it, and then they were like, 'We can't afford to do this.' And they just kept opening things. And now they have the concerts going on again. And everybody's up here like, 'What are you doing?!'"

"Yeah, I don't get it," I said. Yet the week before a friend had offhandedly mentioned that a member of the Arnolds Park city council who owned a huge bar with multiple floors and a rooftop deck was publicly and vehemently against shutting down. When I asked a member of the local Chamber of Commerce what business leaders could do, he said, "the chamber isn't here to regulate business by any means. We're here to support business."

Cheri continued, "We don't get it either. We're like you guys! We get that this is a tourist destination, but one summer for health reasons is not gonna kill the area. I feel like they should listen to people who live here, but unfortunately, it's the tourists that run the area. You know we live here. We pay taxes here. We have a house here. But we don't matter to them."

I shifted in my chair. It was getting late and our conversation was reminding me of Jonathan Metzl's argument that "deeply modern-day American backlash conservatism demands that lower- and middle-class white Americans vote against their own *biological* self-interests as well as their own economic priorities."[16] For example, the GOP quip about promoting "tax breaks" as social policy is something that is widely lauded among card-carrying Republicans. These tax breaks inevitably benefit the wealthy, bolster large corporations, and rarely trickle down.[17] Similarly, unmasking was something that would benefit the wealthy but not the local residents like Cheri who felt forgotten.

"I mean you have people like Butch Parks," Cheri continued. "You know Butch Parks would drown if his businesses didn't run. And considering he now owns Parks Marina, and he owns the Emporium, and he owns the Gardens, like he is a massive running force here. So, yeah. It is the business leaders, it's the city town hall leaders, it's the people that run Arnolds Park, all things. And these people are filthy rich, and they're still saying, 'The financial burden on us would be detrimental if we closed for sixty days to let this COVID thing pass.' They're so worried about the money that they won't do it. So yes. I mean, local money is running everything here, and we have zero say in it."

"So that brings me back to some questions," I said. I went on to ask about the power locals had to change the situation.

"We wanna do something. I think we all wanna do something," Cheri responded. "But I think that people are so powerless to do anything. Like we're all just the basic steel and factory workers here. If we tried to go to the city hall and say we think we should close, I don't think people realize that there's power in numbers. But I also don't think people—and I think you're gonna know what I'm saying from coming from here—people here are afraid to say anything. And unfortunately, this time of year, most of the people who are here right now are here all year. They don't wanna mess up their situation. People just don't wanna rock the boat."

There were significant class differences at play in Okoboji. Cheri explained, "If you try to go tell them, 'We don't want to wear masks. We don't want this.' You're rocking the boat, and rocking the boat would . . ." Cheri trailed off and paused for a minute. I wasn't initially sure who *them* was, but eventually I realized she was talking about wealthier residents in the Iowa Great Lakes. "Okay like if you're coming from the lower spectrum of, you're a factory worker, and we know you're only making like $35,000 a year, and you're rocking the boat against someone that has a house here, [who] makes $3 million [per year], you're never gonna win. Like they're never even gonna listen to you because you don't have the money. Because they don't care. If you're not contributing millions of dollars to Okoboji, they don't care. So . . . ," she trailed off and sighed. "And it's sad but it's seriously true. They [some wealthier residents] just don't care."

"So you think the cops will target you if you rock the boat in what ways?"

"Absolutely. Everybody in Arnolds Park will agree with me if you ask them that." She went on to give a number of examples about how this affected her throughout the summer. Cheri believed that her family was targeted in part because they were lower income. But it also appeared that she felt targeted because coronavirus resistance was imbued in her politics.

"What do you think is going on? Do you think politics is influencing how people are masking or talking about COVID or . . . ," I trailed off, trying to figure out what connections she was conveying to me and why. I thought she was distancing herself from what she perceived to be the elite: wealthy residents, scientists, and the government.

"Yes. I mean when you got the CDC and the World Health Organization saying one thing," Cheri explained, "one day they're saying, 'Only people with symptoms should wear masks.' And then the next day all you see is, 'Everybody should wear masks and we can curve this in, you know we'll have it all gone in a matter of weeks if everybody in America wears a mask.' And it's definitely influencing everybody. And then you've got places like Walmart and Target and Kohl's and Walgreens mandating that people who walk into their store have to have a mask on. But I mean COVID has been here since you know the peak of it in March when we called off schools, and nobody was required to wear a mask. But now all these months into it, now it's a requirement all of a sudden?"

"Why do you think that is?" I asked, realizing that she was grappling with living through a pandemic where the fast pace of policy adaptation sowed some mistrust and confusion. I took a moment to think about how the deeply social response to the pandemic influenced how people thought about masks. Anthropologist Runya Qiaoan reminds us, "Eastern Asian societies, partly due to the memory of SARS, collectively entered a special period swiftly" where "mask-wearing symbolizes knowledge and care." In contrast, in "Western societies, partly due to a century-long lack of personal experience of a severe epidemic," she argued, "mask-wearing symbolizes ignorance and selfishness." She poignantly explains how "the symbolic meaning of masks, instead of being historically and/or culturally given, is reinvented and reinforced due to messages from authorities—governments, media and health experts, in the name of science and value."[18]

"I think it's the media influence," Cheri explained. "I think it's the news scaring everybody and I think it's one person that people think has power saying that if everybody wears a mask, we can get rid of this in a couple weeks. So, everybody's gonna listen and then it takes one person with a powerful voice to stand up and say, 'If you wear a mask, we can get rid of COVID in four weeks.' And then you got everybody saying you know what? Let's jump on that bandwagon! Everybody's just falling in line. Everyone's doing what they're being told to do and I think people honestly need to stop doing it," she paused and I thought maybe the call dropped.

Cheri went on, "You're sitting here like, 'I'm completely healthy. I'm pretty sure I don't have COVID. But you want me to wear a mask? Why?' I think maybe people need to revert the question to them and be like, 'Why do you think I need to have one on? Why do I seem so threatening to you that I need to have a mask on? Because you told me I should?'" She sighed and I could imagine her shaking her head on the other side of the call, or dropping her head into an open palm. "If you go into a Walmart or you go into a restaurant and you don't have [a mask] on, they're like, 'You're part of the problem. You're the reason I might get COVID.'"

I thought for a minute, trying to figure out who was *they*? I think it was scientists, people at risk, or the local elite, who were advocating for public health measures. In many ways, she was angered by the ways people like my family were advocating for stricter masking in public space. She was talking about me.

CHAPTER 10

VACCINE HESITANCY

"YOU SHOULD STAY this year. Just put the girls in school at Spirit Lake," my sister said.

I had just learned in late July that Georgetown University, where I am a professor, was going all virtual—that I would be teaching at least for the next semester completely online. Adam was also working full time from home because researchers at Johns Hopkins University were not allowed in the building (with the exception of those scientists actively working on developing the COVID-19 vaccine). My second grader's class was also completely virtual. My sister had a point.

"Maybe," I said, waffling because I really didn't know what we should do. I was pulled to stay at the Lakes, in the comfort of my family. Yet, many of my students at Georgetown were headed back to campus and I hoped to social distance with those who needed to talk in person: my students lost jobs, family members, and a sense of place, and struggled with overwhelming anxiety. I also felt some uncertainty about sending my kids to my alma mater. I spent so much of the summer talking with people who doubted coronavirus was real and many people resisted masks for the upcoming school year. Would we be safe?

I first started asking about the strong anti-masking stance among some of my yoga friends and quickly realized that mutual friends who were anti-maskers were also anti-vaxxers.[1] I spoke to a woman who knew some of the families driving vaccine hesitancy in the community who I will call Minnie. Minnie explained, "I seriously don't even know how to begin talking about it but like they [the owners of a local business] don't believe in masking. They're anti-vaxxers, which should already tell you how they feel about modern medicine."

I was not surprised to hear Minnie's story, or the frustration she felt. Resistance to vaccination has long cultivated skepticism in what science does and how medicine acts. Vaccine hesitancy was rooted in conspiracy in Britain in the 1880s and came to the United States much later.[2] More recent vaccine hesitancy has been linked to the conspiracy theories promoted by American celebrities that were linked to a debunked 1998 article by Andrew Wakefield and his colleagues published in the *Lancet* that warned the measles vaccine caused autism.[3] This article spurred widespread fear of vaccines. (Although the journal rescinded it a decade later, it caused extraordinary harm and the deaths of multiple children due to measles.[4])

Heidi Larson explains in her book *Stuck: How Vaccine Rumors Start—and Why They Don't Go Away* that the greatest challenge is that it took so long for those working in health and immunization to realize how deeply rooted the beliefs of the doubting public had become. Larson argues "some of these views have hardened to the point of no return, further nursed by the broader societal and political polarization in which the vaccine debates are situated."[5] This polarization is in part behind the emergent trend that the anti-mask group became bound to the anti-vax group: they contend masks are ineffective, cause harm to people's health via hyperventilation or ingesting CO_2, and go against personal freedoms, thereby making them un-American.

"So where did that come from?" I asked Minnie, although I was not surprised by the beliefs of the women she mentioned. I'd grown up with these women; we'd played music together as kids, slugged coffee side-by-side in our teens, and practiced yoga together in the same studio for decades. I had been curious about how they were thinking about coronavirus in part because they are so open about their mistrust of modern medicine on their Facebook feeds. One woman owns a health studio and openly evangelizes her religious, political, and health beliefs through her teaching. A friend said she stopped going there when the owner's fervor for President Trump intensified throughout the Trump presidency. I tried to talk to her but she was too busy with her summer hustle. As the summer waged on, I realized she had un-friended me on Facebook.

"They honestly think that that's the right thing to do," Minnie explained. American sociologist Jennifer Reich wrote a few years ago that "mothers who refuse some or all vaccines access social capital as they gain informational, emotional, and appraisal support from networks for their position and in opposition to those who disapprove."[6] In other words, she found in her work that social power was at the center of vaccine refusal, meaning these women promoted vaccine hesitancy to get something social in return, such as solidarity, respect, or a following.

"I'm not sure they think the vaccines are giving their kids autism," Minnie went on, "but a lot of them were home-schooled. So, they have some basic science not lined up." In some ways, these women fit the anti-vax mold Reich described. She said, "Notably, these women who are racially, educationally, or socioeconomically privileged in some contexts are diminished in others" and "create, promote, and share information to define themselves as experts on their children and on vaccines. These claims of expertise serve to validate their choices and increase their claims to social capital in their networks."[7]

When I heard Minnie talk about these experiences, I couldn't stop thinking about the logic of care. This was in part because she described in detail how an employee of the café was mocked for masking, even when he was doing it to protect his father who was undergoing cancer treatment. She was also teased for masking by a spouse of one of the owners, as he said, "I can't hear you. Maybe it's the mask you're wearing," when she was trying to "do the right thing."

Minnie described how many members of this group of anti-vaxxers and anti-maskers used the debunked CO_2 poisoning mask-argument to garner social power through promoting these beliefs. By posting anti-masking and anti-vaccination posts on Facebook, for example, they carve out a niche of expertise—even when what they post is untrue.

Another way they garnered social power was through outright defiance. For instance, Bethany described how one of these families had their kids run through Walmart when they had COVID-19 to infect others and build immunity in the community. Minnie explained, "They like to bring up how many people die a year from the flu. They're like, there were eight thousand deaths in the US last year from just the flu. So coronavirus isn't taking that big of a toll." Minnie shook her head.

I spoke to another conservative mother earlier in the summer, Jessie, who had had coronavirus amid the spike in June. She expressed an argument for unmasking in order to build immunity that many others I spoke with shared. Jessie explained, "Our take from the beginning was, we wanted it to build our immune systems. We're very, what do you want to say, homeopathic? Vitamins! And we try not to go to the doctor and do all that. So, we wanted it," meaning she wanted to get infected with coronavirus.

I was taken aback by this comment at first. But then I thought back to the chiropractor I spoke to around the same time who suggested vitamin D and sunshine were critical right now to boost one's immune system; she emphasized "eating whole foods, natural things, avoiding the processed sugars, and like all of that stuff." I agreed that eating well amid the pandemic, for a virus that took advantage of a weakened immune system, was critical. Often I prioritize natural remedies first, and for a long time saw a chiropractor for my back (avoiding an orthopedic surgeon to my father's chagrin). In fact, it was massage and sit-ups that helped heal my back—and I avoided the knife. But the narrative about building immunities were different because, although some people with youth and strong immune systems may experience few symptoms, others may unexpectedly die.

Jessie did not dismiss the concern for others who were at risk for serious COVID-19. Jessie went on, "The scary thing I think was when I found out my dad had it because my dad has a compromised immune system. He had some accidents and his immune system might not be the best. So, the scary thing is, if we were to give it to somebody we didn't intend to. And it could be a totally different outcome than what we experienced." I agreed and realized that her understanding of COVID-19 must have been somewhat curtailed before she was infected. Jessie had explained only moments before how she went out to a local bar and wanted to contract COVID-19 to build her immunity and move on with her summer. Perhaps the reality of what it meant only struck when she infected her kids, or perhaps, her father.

I thought again about the chiropractor I spoke to who explained that she wore a mask at work to protect her patients. But then she explained that she never wore a mask otherwise. She even avoided in-person church where they required masks because she did not want to wear one. She carefully described the conspiracy theory about how breathing in CO_2 may damage her health.[8] I saw an increasing number of conspiracy theories and natural remedies for COVID-19 spun on Facebook by other local chiropractors and wondered if their elevated social role in the community may have fostered some of the mistrust in the public health effort.[9]

"What is their solution, just let everyone get it?" I asked Minnie.

"They say, and I quote, 'Our immune systems are strong and we should be able to fight it.' I was like, 'Not everybody, though! Not everybody at all. Like my parents, my grandparents!' I would even argue my forty-year-old colleagues [and] people that are immunocompromised. And every day they post anti-corona propaganda" on Facebook, she alluded, and took a big sigh. "It's embarrassing to read. But they say, 'If you die from it, why are you so afraid of dying? Why are people afraid of dying? When it's your time, it's your time.'"

"So, none of their kids are vaccinated?"

"No. Not a single one," Minnie responded.

DIVERGENT HESITANCIES

I was intrigued by Minnie's story in part because I had just spoken to a woman, whom I will refer to as Maureen, who called herself outright "anti-vax." She became anti-vax after enrolling in a wellness training with the woman Minnie mentioned. The wellness teacher used her studio to evangelize religion, politics, and conspiracy theories, which made me think about how anthropologist EJ Sobo sees vaccine refusals as "crucially generative, in and of themselves, of local in-group relations."[10] This point made me think that Maureen and others were trying—through their anti-vax identity—to carve out a niche to strengthen a small insular social group.

Maureen explained, "I do not trust our government in many, many ways. I don't believe that this is for the people's actual health. And [my belief] pre-dates to when I was pregnant with my son. I did a lot of research on both sides of the vaccine topic. And I guess the stuff that I was finding was disturbing and very swayed to one side. And I started doing more digging on a personal level, kind of what you are doing actually."

"Cool," I said, curious about where she was going.

"So when coronavirus came around my first reaction was like all of this is going to be like the swine flu. You know, it is going to be here and gone, and we are not going to know anyone personally who is infected." She went on to claim the most common conspiracy theories, including the vaccines-cause-autism-cover-up and a belief that coronavirus was made in a laboratory in China— something 40 percent of Americans reported believing, with many people justifying this view by suggesting it appears correct or aligned with their worldview.[11] Maureen's views could be summarized, like other conspiracy theorists, as involving secret plots and influential schemers or agents "working behind the scenes, pulling strings, keeping the truth to themselves because they stand to gain from such undercover intrigue."[12]

In many practical ways, Maureen and the women Minnie described resemble many white women in America who are vaccine hesitant. Reich said, "women who reject vaccines for their children expend significant time and resources managing their children's lives. They describe themselves as able to do so not only through individual immune-promoting practices, like diet and lifestyle, but also by controlling social networks. These mothers see those they believe share their values and lifestyle choices as unlikely to present risk of infection, while evoking unsafe 'outsiders' who carry disease as requiring them to create and laboriously maintain protective barriers."[13] These women tend to be white, with college degrees, left-leaning, and middle class or wealthier.[14]

Yet, they differ from the vaccine hesitant in Okoboji because those in northwest Iowa appear to be more religious and conservative than the vaccine-hesitant mothers Reich wrote about. In some ways, their vaccine hesitancy entwines socio-spiritual views on personal connections with the body, God, politics, and their insular community through which they navigate belief, power, and white privilege. For instance, Jessie told me she did not fear coronavirus because "we know where we're going when we die. We put our trust in God. There's no fear." This was also a common narrative among some chiropractors in town, as well as the broader wellness community. Another central feature for many people was their support for President Trump, as many conveyed him as a messianic figure, anointed by God.[15] These beliefs were intensified through a type of Charismatic Christianity that many people in this group practiced (where people directly connect to the Holy Spirit).[16] Referring to coronavirus beliefs, written on a local church website is this suggestion: "Please respect others and be kind to those who have different ideas or precautions than you."[17]

In contrast, many white evangelical men conveyed another type of vaccine hesitancy that became central to COVID-vaccine resistance in Okoboji and the United States more broadly. Many white men believe resisting the vaccine is a "freedom" or "civil liberties" issue.[18] A Pew Research Center study found that partisan differences were increasingly observed to influence vaccine intent, with Republicans much less likely to say they planned to get vaccinated. Much of this hesitancy was associated with "trust in the vaccine research and development process."[19] For instance, National Public Radio quoted a man who said, "My fear of the vaccine is more than my fear of getting the illness."[20] Some of this distrust could have been overcome with President Trump making a show of getting the vaccine. However, he chose to do so in private. In an article titled "White Evangelical Resistance Is Obstacle in Vaccine Effort," Elizabeth Dias and Ruth Graham said, "The sheer size of the community poses a major problem for the country's ability to recover from a pandemic that has resulted in the deaths of half a million Americans. And evangelical ideas and instincts have a way of spreading, even internationally."[21]

"It is a whole thing, that operation 2021, I think." It took me a minute to realize that Maureen was speaking about conspiracy theories purported by pro-Trump conspiracy theorist QAnon that aligned COVID-19 with global population control.[22] Maureen went on to describe this eugenic conspiracy theory, bringing health, racial, and climate crises together. She named COVID, George Floyd, and heat as combined government conspiracies to reduce population.

She later followed up with me to share several unrelated text messages on these conspiracies. She also sent me a list of forty imagined facts she collected about vaccines. I started looking them up, one after one, and had a difficult time following the logic.

These conspiracy theories and in-group social pressures that fuel vaccine hesitancy among white people differ in meaningful ways when compared to what causes vaccine hesitancy among communities of color. For instance, many Black Americans describe anti-Black state violence in America that fuels medical racism, reinforcing mistrust and causing neglect, harm, and fear among Black mothers over generations, as central to vaccine hesitancy.[23] These systemic issues differ in meaningful ways from reasons of culture, belief, and social power that have been cited among many white evangelical men and white women on both the left and right.

Maureen and I finished our conversation with her musing, "I'm very tolerant obviously. What you choose to do to keep your child safe in your own beliefs is like your thing." This made me think again about the logics of choice versus the logics of care, where vaccination was essentially a tool to care for others as opposed to the self. But complex histories of trust and mistrust in the government and corporate interests could not be dislodged from mistrusting Americans' realities. In many ways, vaccine hesitancy has been weaponized by some as a social and political tool to garner social status, personal legitimacy, and political power at the expense of other people's health.[24] This is not unlike anti-maskers who fueled a national debate and culture war around wearing a mask to keep others safe; in this case, the *mask* was weaponized and used as a social tool to control people's behavior, despite their health risk.

Months later I heard that a physician in Zach's practice actively deterred patients from getting the COVID-19 vaccine, arguing that, based on a circulating conspiracy theory, the vaccine would change your DNA.[25] I heard from a patient that they were shocked to receive this advice, and many people were flabbergasted that the barrage of misinformation carried on for so long.[26] Patients reported to Avera that this physician advised them against taking the vaccine because it would manipulate their DNA. Soon after, he left the practice, but the official reasons for leaving remain unclear. Protesters gathered a couple times in the spring outside the hospital to promote false ideas that the vaccines are more deadly than COVID-19, trying to influence a few more people to embrace vaccine hesitancy.

CHAPTER 11

SCHOOL BOARD

THE GREAT PLAINS are known for their extreme temperatures and winds. In the winter the air is so cold your fingers freeze, while the bright sun gives you a sunburn and the winds whip you off your feet. In July, the sun is so hot and dry that you need to be near water to cool off. Often by the end of July the bright sun recedes some, the temperatures come back down to the eighties, and the crowds in Okoboji thin. People are getting ready to return to school.

Sitting on a bench at Speier Park, watching my daughters loft tennis balls over the net, I spoke to a childhood friend who I call Kristin. As I sat there, I thought about how thirty years before, we had been lofting tennis balls over the same nets, and out of the park. Although a line of century-old trees protects you from the hot sun by the playground, the area around the courts has been completely cleared. Sweat dripped down my back as we spoke.

It was a somewhat awkward conversation. I had reached out to her early upon my arrival home to set up an interview. Usually we get together for a glass of wine or a playdate with the kids to catch up after the school year. She is one of my oldest friends who I still stay in touch with when I'm home. At first, I was surprised by Kristin's steadfast resistance: *I am not interested in participating in research!* I didn't understand this response for a long time, in part because she was a retired nurse practitioner with young children the ages of my girls. I knew she was careful about where she went with her kids, although I had observed many unmasked photos on social media and run into her eating out during my one lunch out for an interview. She is conservative, like the rest of the Spirit Lake School Board. But as a medical professional, she was clearly concerned about the virus.

I realized over the course of the summer that her resistance to speaking with me was simply because she is politically savvy. Later she told me that the school board members had made up their minds in April about how they felt about masking. She could not compromise her position as the one person who was advocating for stricter public health recommendations by speaking openly with me. In early August, when I attended two open forums about returning to school—when masking was hotly debated and haphazardly supported—it was clear where she stood. She was speaking from a position of scientific authority, while the rest of the school board was not. She feared an interview, even conducted confidentially, would undermine her public health advocacy within the local schools.

Kristin maintained a laissez faire attitude about coronavirus on Facebook early in the summer, but was the only school board member to post about masking. Her post showed her kids at Arnolds Park Amusement Park, where masking was mandatory. The amusement park had closed down in June for several weeks to regroup and introduce stringent masking, cleaning, and social distancing protocols. My father had been on the park's board for a couple decades and we had heard that the administration was committed to enforcing public health measures there. In many ways, the park, with its century-old wooden roller coaster, implemented the best public health protocols in town. It was only rivaled by its neighbor, the Nutty Bar Stand. The Nutty Bar Stand was owned by a nurse who lost no time meeting with and collaboratively setting up ground rules for her staff of teenage ice-cream scoopers and establishing social distancing protocol for customers. The Nutty Bar Stand plastered big red circles to the floor so customers knew where to stand, set up multiple hand sanitizer stations, implemented a mask mandate, and removed seating. There was a line—though a socially distanced one (some of the time)—out the door throughout the summer.

As you ride up the first hill of the roller coaster at Arnolds Park, a sign says, "Point of No Return!" This was an apt metaphor for the school board meetings in early August, when their decisions would shape the rest of the year for many families. On Friday, July 17, Governor Kim Reynolds ordered in a proclamation, "Students learn best when they're in school. For all of the wonders of online and distanced learning—and it does play a role—it's not a replacement for in-person classes. We also can't forget the critical role that our schools play in addressing inequities for our most vulnerable student populations."[1]

It was hard to disagree with this statement. As a mother of a second grader and pre-kindergartener, there was nothing that I wanted more than for my children to be in school in a safe and supportive environment.

Reynolds went on, "I know this is not going to be easy, I know it's going to require some changes to how things are done in the classroom. But given the importance of education to our children and the people of Iowa, we owe it to them to just roll up our sleeves and get our schools back up and running safely and effectively."[2]

This proclamation was one of the only state-wide policies the governor implemented for coronavirus. Yet, again, Governor Reynolds left it up to local authorities to determine what worked best for community health and safety. In part, relegating power to the local level made sense, because rural towns had very different exposures and risks for coronavirus when compared to urban centers like Des Moines and Cedar Rapids. But it also created a hugely contested space for communities to spar over hot-button topics like masking.

CORONA-COASTER

The schools had shut down on March 16, 2020, and most families and educators were looking forward to them opening up in August for the following school year. Yet the uncertainty of what the school year would look like in July stressed many educators in the area. I connected with teachers from each of the three school districts to learn how they were thinking about the likelihood of in-person school plans. I asked one teacher (who I will call Mary), "How are you feeling about them being open completely?"

Mary replied, "Have you heard the term *corona-coaster*?"

I smiled, thinking about the old wooden roller coaster and the emotional ride we had been on for several months. "I have actually not heard that term but I love that."

"It is perfect really because it is how I've lived since March basically, and I'm still that way right now. But I'm a big-time overthinker and I always have a little health anxicty anyway," Mary explained. "There are some mornings that I get up and [my son] is going to football workouts. He was in baseball—having the normalcy of baseball, although I was anxious about it at first, it kind of saved my summer. And so I think, and [my son] is so funny, bless his heart, he had to counsel his mom a lot this summer. So he just told me today, 'Mom, honestly, once you get into school, it will all just be normal again. It will be fine.' Now there is also the critical thinker in me that thinks: but will it? So, there is that corona-coaster that I just want it to be normal and I want to get back into it. I feel like our district, and maybe I'm wrong, but I feel like that, because of our area [politics], our district is going to go full in, no masks. I think they will be recommended but not required. I could be wrong. I've been surprised in the past with things. But I feel that, I don't think we are going to follow a lot of anything. And hopefully we are in an area [that is low risk], although it is a tourist area but rural enough. You know it is not like New York City or something. We are able to get through it."

The anxiety this teacher communicated came out in myriad ways across my interviews with teachers, counselors, nurses, and parents in the school system. For example, I spoke to another teacher and his wife (I'll call them Rob and Raina), who were lifelong Republicans and spoke freely about their disdain for President Trump's handling of the pandemic. They closely tracked the Johns Hopkins Coronavirus Resource Center, which tallied numbers in each state and county.

I asked, "How do you think the governor has done managing the pandemic?"

"At first great," Rob said.

Raina interjected, "It seems like everybody was, you know, doing what they needed to do at first, like we were all in this together. Then I did sense a difference and change. I don't know how far we got into it, but it seemed like once we started, once the economy started getting really bad, stuff started to seem to change."

"Yeah, she had pressure from Trump or whoever," Rob continued, "to get those meat-packing plants in line and keep the production up, and she started taking her hands off the steering wheel and let locals take over."

"Each county," said Raina.

"An each county kind of thing," Rob confirmed.

"It seemed like she changed a little bit that way about getting the economy back to where it was working again."

"And just recently the *Des Moines Register* put out an article about schools. They are not going to be having a lot of requirements for school! They are going to leave it up to the local officials to take over. And, again, they don't want blame on their back is what I'm guessing."

I interjected, "You think that is it?"

"I don't know," Rob said. "It has come down to the individuals, the parents to [decide to] send their kids back to school or not. And I think the other states were having the option of hybrid if they could send their kids back or they could do 100 percent online. That works for nonworking families."

"Yeah," Raina agreed.

Although Rob and Raina lived on a farm, with plenty of land for their children to run, play, camp, and be outside, they still faced social stress around coronavirus. Their teenager was invited to participate in softball, but they chose not to participate because, as Rob explained, "we didn't agree with not sanitizing the equipment."

I eventually shifted our conversation back to politics because Rob had mentioned how frustrated he was with Trump's handling of coronavirus. I asked, "What do you think about Trump and national politics? How has that affected how you think about it?"

"He is a joke," Rob answered. "I mean, at first he was following his advisory committee. Then he was starting to go off the rails and fire people and kind of go against what Fauci was saying. I got way more respect for Fauci than Trump."

"He should have run for president," I joked.

"Yeah!" Raina agreed.

"Yeah, we have our state officials that are just listening to Trump and he has nothing to do with the medical community, he has no idea what is going on," Rob explained.

"I really thought it was crazy to hear him say we shouldn't be testing and that if we don't test, we don't know," Raina said.

"Our numbers would go down!" Rob joked.

"If you test then that means the numbers go up. I just had trouble listening to that."

Rob continued, "But I thought at first he was doing a good job with his briefings and then just after a few weeks of going through it, stuff started to unravel, especially when they started talking about firing Dr. Fauci. I don't know what was going on!"

"Again, I think it comes down to economics. I think [Trump] wants his numbers to be up to make him look good," Raina suggested. I thought about how this contrasted with how Trump thought testing "makes us look bad" and argued against more testing because he didn't want "higher numbers."[3]

"Yeah, I just lost trust in him," Rob said. "I didn't have any faith in him anymore after that because it is like: are you choosing the economy over people's lives or how do you balance that? I was looking for balance."

"Did you support him before the pandemic?" I asked.

"I did, yeah," said Rob.

"I was in the middle," Raina replied. "I'm an independent so I think I did vote for him because at the time I didn't want to vote for Hillary. I think he has done a good job with the economy. I will say I think he does well as far as that stuff goes."

"He plays games and he takes risks at other people's expense though," Rob interjected. "He doesn't always think about who he is hurting."

"I don't really like some of the . . . ," Raina paused and thought a minute. "I don't like him as a person, the way he treats people, the things he says."

"No," Rob said sternly. And from his face, I could see that he meant it.

"So, no, I don't like that about him," Raina concluded.

"Do you think it has an influence on how you are going to vote or not?"

"What he has done with the pandemic," Raina responded. "I won't say the pandemic is going to decide my voting for him. I would say it is just his personality that will help me decide. I don't know who I'm going to vote for yet. I haven't found a good candidate yet."

Teachers like Rob and Mary provided a critical story for thinking about how educators and parents perceived school reopening. On the one hand, they wanted their children to resume normal life. On the other, they knew the risks their families faced and how little power they had to determine what would happen with regard to administrative decisions. They recognized that the governor was closely aligned with the president. Every educator I spoke to was worried about the fact that the governor demanded a full return to school without, in their view, adequate support mechanisms for schools to bring students back safely.

When I asked a retired teacher (who I will call Susie) what she thought about Governor Reynolds's return-to-school plan, Susie explained, "Oh you know, I liked her at the beginning but I guess there are two sides. If she told the schools what to do, then they would be mad, they would say, 'where is our local control?' If instead, she didn't tell them what to do, and now they are saying, 'where is the guidance?' So, it's half one, half the other. And at the same point I do think that each school district has to make their own decision for their own community. Because what we are doing in Spirit Lake might be totally different from what they are doing in Des Moines. I guess it is up to local control."

Susie went on to focus on Dr. David Smith, the superintendent for the Spirit Lake Community School District. "Who is the one that should make that decision? Should it be Dr. Smith? Should it be school board members? And I think now that the school board [members] are the ones. Because they are the ones that should be blamed if it doesn't go right. It is the school board because that is who everybody hired [in the local election]. So, I'm hoping that [Kristin—my friend who was the only nurse on the school board], and the others are reading what educators are saying, what doctors are saying."

Nearly everyone I spoke to wanted the children to return to school. Many cited the socioeconomic inequalities emerging because of being out of school. Community members were worried about kids getting enough nutritious food when they missed school lunch. They were also worried about who was watching children when parents had to work. Working families and single mothers were struggling the most.

At the same time, many teachers expressed concern about who held the power to determine what public health prevention modes would be put in place. With local

leadership in charge, would they follow science and implement public health recommendations? Would they let partisan politics lead? The community had great uncertainty
around how the school board would vote to protect the
public's health: Would the school board require students
to mask? How could the teachers get a face shield? Do
teachers have to get close to students? Could the teachers
install their own Plexiglas around each desk? One teacher
said her husband could build Plexiglas dividers for each
desk in her classroom. But she said he could not do that
for everyone. How do you do science labs?—sometimes
you have to get close to look into a microscope. Another
teacher was worried about bending down to help students
with homework. What would social distancing mean in
the classroom?

Yet the community was utterly divided. While most
people I spoke to wanted public health measures like masking in place in schools, many others did not. *We will not
send our children to schools in masks!* This was expressed
by some parents of children with disabilities who were
very concerned about how their children would handle
masking. But many others, like Maureen and Jessie (and
people across the nation), spewed conspiracy theories
such as "masks cause harm from carbon dioxide!" Mostly,
people felt that masking should be a choice that each family
made independently. Like vaccinations, people thought
families should be able to opt out of masking because of
personal beliefs. These beliefs played out in real ways on
the school board, revealing a powerful invocation of what

was perceived as personal choice over personal responsibility in the context of learning environments.

SUPERINTENDENT

I followed the Spirit Lake School District planning closely because my niece and nephew were enrolled, and the planning was a constant discussion at our house. I completed K–12 at the public school in Spirit Lake, so I know the buildings and community well, although they have modified the buildings over the course of the twenty years since I'd left. Even still, I am constantly hearing about school politics from my mother, who has volunteered in the guidance office, tutoring students in math for the past thirty years.

When Spirit Lake initially decided to go back to school, they were very clear that the administration would meet the six feet social distancing regulation advocated by the CDC. This meant that the administration would make every effort to keep students six feet apart at all times. The superintendent went to extremes to do this with a process of school renovations, by moving walls and renting space off campus for additional classrooms. Spirit Lake's ability to achieve these physical changes to the school buildings was in part due to the money in the district. The high school was built in 1960 and has had major renovations in the past decade (including a new theatre and classrooms). The elementary school was built in 1980, and the middle school was built in 1990. I remember how cold it was in the double-wide trailer that we used as a classroom during the elementary school remodel. I was in Mrs. Tibben's fourth grade classroom—you could hear the wind outside the thin walls.

Where and how to move walls and rearrange classrooms was a central focus of the Spirit Lake School Board's open forum working group on August 3, 2020. Zach and I drove together: he was worried about the meeting because his public health colleagues were frustrated after meeting with the administration earlier that day. We got in the car and Zach said, "It's in the administrative building. We should be able to slip right in." Zach and I arrived just on time, and the room was already full of twenty other people: mostly parents, educators, and coaches.

Half of us were in masks, and half were not. The superintendent, associate administrator, lawyer, and six school board members sat shoulder-to-shoulder around a small table in a small room. None of the board members wore masks. Everyone seemed a bit twitchy.

The superintendent, Dr. Smith, opened the meeting with a five-minute monologue about uncertainty. He said, "You know the name of the game is communication. But with that said, glad we had [the renovations] moving faster with the detail work. We said a lot of back-to-school, face-to-face, that was a really great decision. But a lot of the details, as you know schools have come out and said, 'hey, we are going to go online here, and the governor says this and some change happens.' So there is some frustration throughout the state. So the school administration and parents, every week that goes by, we get a little bit more guidance. So even though you might receive some complaints or whatever, [people saying,] 'hey we need all of these details right now!,' honestly it is not even realistic because it could possibly change. So hang in there with that and know that we are okay. Everybody knows we have to come to school. The teachers know they have to educate the kids. We will be cleaning. You know there are questions about masks. I think that is probably the biggest issue and I've put that at the end of the list here to talk about, because I think that is going to require most of the discussion."

Dr. Smith spent the next fifteen minutes talking. He discussed challenges the administration faced, like who will support the bus driver and where they would rent extra space to make sure desks could be spaced six feet apart. He indicated that the administration consulted with public health officials and realized there was little wiggle room around the six feet and fifteen minutes of indoor contact rules.

He explained, "I am just really trying to understand details about what we should be focused on as a school perspective. [We are] trying to balance that with the governor. And we heard the governor talk about six feet, fifteen minutes, and all of that. And then you hear a lot about masks and all of that. Our discussion today is just on a couple of questions. But I wanted to talk first on cleaning."

Dr. Smith went on to explain the intricacies of what would be cleaned in classrooms and when. Who would clean and how they would do it. He explained that the administration would move walls to expand classrooms.

All elementary school classrooms were expanded, and some middle school classes were moved off site. They were able to make sure all desks in every class were six feet apart. Many board members were delighted because most classrooms had a door that opened outside, so they could leave that door ajar when the weather was nice. The possibility of having airflow was a relief. They were certain the desks could be spaced apart six feet. Many were uncertain about how to handle the bus: would there be an extra teacher available to make sure kids stayed in line? Also, how do we space out movement between classes to make hallways less packed? The only thing that the members of the school board were not clear about was masks.

DISREGARD OF EXPERTISE

Although the school board said they were relying on the recommendations of public health advisors, their reliance on public health recommendations seemed to be a farce. I had also spoken to public health advisors and local physicians who were frustrated by how the superintendent handled (or, in their opinion, disregarded) their guidance. In some ways, the public health team described the administration's behavior as aggressive and probing for less stringent measures. I heard this from five different people, but I'll focus on one person's response.

A public health official from the hospital explained, "It was like a firing squad. It was just unfair what they did. [pause] We were going to have it at the hospital. And then the night before the meeting (and it was Monday), so Sunday night at like 8:45, they sent an email, [saying a] 'little change of plans. Dr. Smith is going to be there. And [the athletic director] is going to be there. And it's going to be at the school.' So [we] moved it to the school and then we got there and then all the principals were there. It was seven [people from the school] against two [people from the hospital], and it felt that way. And then we just immediately started getting railed with questions and very specific scenarios of clearly, clearly trying to skirt the rules."

The advisor went on, "The focus wasn't so much on reducing transmission as it was about reducing the burden of contact tracing.[4] And so, it was like, well, what if we keep someone together for fourteen minutes and thirty seconds and then they run away? And we were like, *no*. And then just trying to figure out scenarios for when they could take masks off. And they kept trying to ask the same question over and over and over and over and over and over and over again to try and get us to contradict ourselves and contradict each other. So it was a competitive environment for sure."

I found the political delicacy around these decisions fascinating. Small towns create special situations where people talk on and off the record. While social networks influence most political decision-making, social ties in small towns go back generations. In this case, two brothers, a school administrator and the top medical advisor to the school district, were involved in negotiating public health recommendations between the school and hospital. In the long run, I imagine their relationship played a role in the school district's eventual adoption of stricter masking measures.

Perhaps they sat down and discussed the implications of mask-avoidance and came up with a plan to enact smarter public health protocol from behind the scenes. But there may be other factors that played a role in the final decision, which I will explain soon. What many perceived as flippancy around these public health measures in the open forum and hostility in the closed-door meeting were likely associated with the superintendent, according to the people I interviewed. Some people found him domineering.

Susie talked about the superintendent's overbearing presence at length. "I can't believe the school board meetings take half an hour! Sure is quick and they get out. We don't get to hear what the school members think!" We were sitting on a park bench, masked, and looking out over East Lake Okoboji, a five-minute jog from Big Spirit Lake and the spillway. In 1993, we spent hours upon hours at the spillway filling sandbags for people in the community whose houses flooded during the rainy summer. The community came together and helped each other. I reflected on how central that was to how I remember the community of my childhood.

Susie went on, "I think the school board, they give the authority to Dr. Smith and to the principals and all that. But they are the governing body of the school!"

My contact from the hospital went on to explain the confrontation between public health and the school administration: "I mean, it was to get the soundbite that they wanted. They wanted a rubber stamp from public health to say in some snippet you can take your masks off in this scenario. And they kept trying to really push the boundaries and say, well, we're going to remove the walls in the elementary school and we'll promise that they'll be six feet apart all the time. It was like, you know, fifteen minutes. I mean, I've been talking with epidemiologists. Fifteen minutes is not a magic number. It's just not. I mean, you can get it in fifteen seconds if you're in the right situation. That number is for the back-end contact tracing and having some kind of guideline of where to start, who to trace. But you can't proactively be like 'oh! thirteen minutes and fifty-six seconds, we're good.' And that is how they're treating it. That is how they're doing it but that doesn't work. But what is a magic number? At least what they feel is slightly magical. Is that six feet. So distance does matter. But then I just kept trying to say, layering is the most important thing you can be doing right now." I thought for a minute about how smart that concept was: layering. But rarely had I heard it in discussions about returning to school. My contact continued, "Why would you only choose one safeguard when you can do three? Why wouldn't you layer on distancing with masking with hand hygiene?"

The public health official continued, "Because the more you do, the more likely you are to mitigate transmission. It breaks down to the fact that they're really frustrated that even if kids are both masked, then you find that one is positive, they still are going to be quarantined because it's not PPE. And so, they're like, well, then why mask? Why mask if it's not going to take away the contact tracing and the quarantine? So, and I understand it's extremely frustrating to have one kid lead to a domino effect of like fifty kids out like that. That is horrible, especially from an administrative standpoint. But the game isn't about finding loopholes and literally trying to game the system. The game is trying to keep as many people safe as possible and the school open in a safe way. So, Okoboji's [leadership has] been amazing."

I already knew Okoboji's high school principal's leadership around masking was aligned with what the public health team was advising. I knew where he stood in part from conversations with Zach but mostly because the care this principal was taking in listening to teachers and the community came up frequently when I spoke with teachers, counselors, and administrators from Okoboji—many of whom were my classmates growing up in Spirit Lake schools. One employee at Okoboji schools, who I call Derek, said, "I think it is silly to not be requiring masks."

Derek went on, "And my personal view has changed a lot over the course of this [pandemic] on that. But the way I see it is, if wearing a piece of fabric over my face might help somebody's ninety-six-year-old father . . ." Derek paused for a minute and a soft expression came over his face. "We had a father of a current student die. And it just seems like such a silly little thing [to have to debate about masks]. But our [school] board spent three hours discussing the word 'recommend' versus 'require.'"

"That is why I thought it was an interesting meeting," I said, referring to the Spirit Lake meeting that I had just attended the day before.

"And knowing the dynamics of the Spirit Lake board," Derek said, "you have got board members there that are connected to the medical field like [Kristin]. And then you have board members there that are very business people."

"Is that [Shane]?" I bought insurance from him for my first car, so I had met with him several times but didn't know him well.

"Yeah. And I see they keep pushing the decision. They keep kicking the can down the road a little bit and I get it. They don't want to make the decision too early. I get that things change. But if our board members' meeting was any indication, then they are in for a big shock when they have to [make the decision]. It was such a bad one here on Wednesday."

"So, you guys eventually decided to recommend masks right against the school recommendation?" I asked.

"Yeah," Derek replied. "So, the admin team had put together a thirty-two-point plan, with everything from what is lunch going to look like to masks. And we presented this to the board last Wednesday and they loved it. The only thing literally, the only topic of conversation at least in the past week's meeting, was masks. And it was heated, you know, all the meetings are heated. I don't envy them right now. Especially in this part of the state. It is definitely a unique thing up here as opposed to other parts of the state because of the political landscape up here. I mean, because frankly, there is going to be a Trump boat rally this weekend. It is just going to be huge on West Lake. It has become political. You know what I mean? It just has."

I had heard about the Trump boat parade. This was just one of the unreal experiences that was happening this summer. In Okoboji, protest was happening on the lake itself. (Although this was not unique in itself—boat protests or celebrations were happening throughout Trump's presidency around the nation.)

After discussing leadership in education, Derek continued, "A couple of weeks ago [Brian Downing, the Okoboji High School principal] put a post on his personal Facebook [page] wearing a mask and just kind of outlining, *I'm choosing to wear it in public spaces, even though I'm not personally afraid of getting the virus.*" Brian posted a picture of himself in a mask in front of an Okoboji Pioneers sign, demonstrating his allegiance to the school. But he posted this support for masking amid a heated debate about sending kids back to school with a mask mandate versus a mask recommendation. The notion that masks would be mandated made some families so furious they threatened to homeschool their children. Brian posted:

> I have avoided joining in this discussion because it, like seemingly everything else in the world, has become political but the Coronavirus took away my favorite three months of last school year and now threatens the start of the next one. It has also sickened several of my personal acquaintances and taken the life of a wonderful local leader, father, and husband.
>
> I have a very public role and, good or bad, my actions are noticed on a local level. This brings a responsibility to model the actions I believe are in the best interests of our school and community.
>
> For all these reasons, I wear a mask.
>
> I want to go to school and I want to see every student and staff member there every day. So I wear a mask.

I care about the wellbeing of those around me and the wellbeing of their loved ones. So I wear a mask.

I believe in science and, when given the opportunity to protect others at nothing more than a slight discomfort or inconvenience to myself, I take that opportunity. So I wear a mask.

I don't wear it to make a political statement. I don't wear it to start a debate. I don't wear it because it is comfortable (although it's really not that bad.) I don't even wear it to protect myself.

I wear it because the science tells me it could help keep others from getting sick. I wear it because I want to go to work. I wear it because I want my kids to go to school this year and run cross-country and swim and play music. I wear it because I care about my community.

I wear it because others are watching me.

(I am smiling by the way.)[5]

I did not find this post shocking. Instead, I found it incredibly warm and exactly what I would expect a community leader to post in July when the community was discussing going back to school amid a global pandemic. What was shocking was the vitriol he received in response.

One parent responded to this post very charged up. I was curious immediately about this parent's long response, as well as their profile photo, which showed a child on a boat with a "Trump 2020: No More Bullshit!" flag in the background. This individual wrote:

Let's look at the facts in our country. There are minimal positive tests. No children! This is insanity. We need to be LIONS! Not sheep. Open our school! I implore you to advocate No masks! We have special needs children in MY family that will not/cannot wear a mask. Stop the fear mongering! If the virus was so bad why did our summer sports happen? No spikes after 1000's of people hear [*sic*] on the 4th of July. Kids under 18 are not the spreaders of this!!! I am absolutely ashamed by your post. Our children are suffering. I know this first hand!!!! I AM going to be the voice of reason in this community. You actually are taking a stance when many many doctors do not agree with what you are saying. My 4 children will take the HIPPA [*sic*] mask exception!!! You must resign immediately!! And your [*sic*] "only wearing it because people are watching me" so that means, you hold no truth to what you are saying.

The individual then continued with,

I'm so fundamentally disturbed by this post! [Referring still to Brian]. He's a leader and a teacher! He is supposed to lead impartially! This is wrong on all levels. I have 4 children that will go to [school] and not ONE will keep the mask on. It's wrong, just wrong! What do I do with my 2 special needs kids? Get phone calls every day about how they were disrupting the class bc they couldn't keep it on? Hell no, I have a job also and won't accept this! It's not transmitted by kids, if you are sick or scared stay the heck home, homeschool! As for the teachers who are scared, stay home! He looks NOT happy, he's NOT smiling, and his last sentence states, "I wear it because others are watching me". Proof he hates it and is only wearing to make a state-

ment. Look at your face in the pic. You look miserable!!!!!!!
Imagine the kids! Read your oath Brian!!!!!!!!!! Read
it!!!!!!!!!! Be impartial!!!!!!! Very very upset right now!
I agree what's best for the kids! Always! This is not!!!!!! [6]

This individual sent a private message to Brian to apologize later. When I spoke with him a couple weeks after the incident, he was frustrated but also sympathetic. He was mostly worried about the politics the students would face because their parents were so fired up—on both sides. Most everyone concerned about masking thought masking was a farce at best and caused harm to kids by making them ingest carbon dioxide at worst. There was no evidence for these claims. They'd read it on Facebook.

Reflecting on this post, Derek said, "I mean, full disclosure: the [people who attacked Brian] are the organizers of the Trump boat rally. And they were just saying how terrible leadership is and how [teachers are] clearly going to be biased against some kids whose parents don't want them to wear them. I mean they were just making things up. And that is why I don't envy the board members because, you know, a school doesn't exist in a vacuum. We exist in a political climate. And I think that Iowa by several measures, we are the only state that I understand is requiring in-person school and doesn't have a mask mandate." Derek shook his head.

"A couple of days ago, there were five. I think now there are four?" I asked.

"And I haven't fact checked it but I saw a list of five states that are requiring in-person school," Derek replied.

I double checked and in August there were four states with state-ordered in-person instruction: Iowa, Missouri, Arkansas, and Texas. By September Missouri removed the mandate; however, Florida shifted to mandate in-person instruction the same month.[7]

Derek continued, "And you put together in-person school plus no [mask] mandate—it seems to maybe just be Iowa. And this is the environment that these board members are having to try and make decisions in. In the board meeting, we talked for three hours about the word [mandate]. And our recommendation was not full masks all day. There are lots of schools that are doing that. We were trying to find a compromise, Emily, because we know where we live and we know that if we went in and said eight-to-three, we are going to require masks, there was no way that was going to happen."

I found it so interesting how every detail about masks was constantly negotiated. It seemed to me that it would be simple for Governor Reynolds to mandate masks in schools and save administrators, teachers, and parents a great deal of stress. I also remembered back to what the local lawyer had told me: unless you enforce the mandate, it's not practical. I wondered if there was too much local dissent, from the superintendent to local parents, to enforce a mandate.

Derek continued, "So, we tried to say there are some situations that are going to be required. We recommend not all day. We are going to require [masking] when social distancing is at its least: so passing time in the hallways, group work. Whenever basically you are not sitting in straight rows at least three feet apart, you know what I mean? And I think we are all starting to use that three-foot rule now because we don't like the six-foot rule. It doesn't mean anything," he stated, referring to the social distancing guidelines, which felt so arbitrary.

He concluded, "These are the only areas that we require their use and the rest would be recommended. And the board said no on a three to two vote. The board president was very adamant," Derek explained. "So, we are highly recommended—whatever highly means. Ultimately, it comes down to: is there going to be a fine if you don't follow it or not? And the answer is no. Spencer and Estherville have both required masks. Lake Park is recommending just like we are. And then we will wait and see where Spirit Lake ends up."

I was also very interested in how the Spirit Lake school board members would talk about masks. Spencer and Estherville *required* masks, although they reside in counties that were much stricter in public health enforcement throughout the summer. Okoboji and Lake Park—both in Dickinson County—were *recommending* masks. This policy was similar to how businesses had recommended people wear masks throughout the one hundred days of summer. It was clear that a recommendation in the tourist region resulted in few people wearing masks in public. As I sat on the edge of my seat, waiting for the school board working group discussion in Spirit Lake to lay their cards on the table, I thought, Would they follow suit?

CHAPTER 12

CONTESTED

WHEN THE SPIRIT Lake School Board working group eventually turned to masks, each person had prepared notes. Kristin told me later that all board members had made up their minds in April. There was no way to change how they would vote.

Shane, a middle-aged insurance agent who was dressed nicely in a button-down shirt and dress pants, started with an argument of liberty and personal freedoms. He stated, "I have just been stewing over it and I have a hard time dictating to people in general. The five of us telling kids how to act. On the flip side, when people decide what to do, we have to ask the community too. That's their personal decision. We need to respect, understand. We are a public institution and there are things we have to take care. We have to be super flexible with one decision or another. This is not one decision. Those are just my thoughts."

I turned to Zach and whispered, "But isn't that their job? Aren't they supposed to decide what's best for your community?"

Next was Kristin. "I agree with you, especially on personal choice and personal freedoms. But when I think of our students, especially nine through twelfth [grade], we don't give them a choice to come to school. Really, we mandate! It's law that they come to school. And I think that is where I have a difficult time around this. When we wanted to run for the school board, making choices about our children's health is one thing that really matters. It is the last thing I think about when I fall asleep and the first thing when I wake up. And it is consuming everyone in this room. It has been very difficult. And so, when I think of those students that we require them to come to school, I want to make sure that we get it right."

Kristin sat, poised, in a smart black dress with styled hair, next to Dr. Smith, in a suit. She looked around the room, and continued, "I care deeply that we protect [the children] and that is why I feel more comfortable with everyone wearing masks. I know it is not a popular choice and it goes against my own personal views and it does conflict with personal freedoms, personal choice, and personal responsibility. But at the end of the day, I just want to make sure that I have a strong feeling that we really get this right. And one way is protecting wearing masks. They are imperfect; they are not 100 percent protective, but if it is something that will prevent the spread, particularly from ninth through twelfth [grades]."

Kristin took a breath and went on, "I am less supportive of mandating masks for elementary. I think small kids, PK through middle school, is kind of a grey area for me, I'm not sure. I don't think they understand why they need to wear them. This is coming from my own five-, six-, and eight-year-olds. The longest they have been able to wear them is one hour and I've been trying, lots of bribes! The Sugar Shack!" she jibed. The room burst into laughter, with the reminder of the summer sweets cutting the tension.

She went on, "They are good for maybe forty-five minutes, then they can't. Again, they don't understand how you don't touch your mouth, you know? And I think that is an unreasonable burden to put on those teachers on top of educating and getting everybody back to where we were early in March. Leave your mask on! Put your mask on! That is why I'm not in favor for the lower levels mandating masks. Where I see it more of an issue in the nine through twelve and the staff, as well. Again, I know my choice, and I've heard from everybody across the spectrum. And that is where I fall in the minority."

Even though Kristin was the only one who put forth a pro-masking argument, I was really glad to hear it. Zach breathed out slowly as she spoke. He said in the car that he knew Kristin would be supportive of some measures for public health recommendations. Although he was hoping for universal masking, this support was helpful.

SPEAKING FOR POPULAR BELIEF

After Kristin's defense of masking, the president of the school board, Sharon, spoke. "So, if I had to vote today based on what I'm looking at right there," Sharon looked up at a chart of cases that had been posted by the county supervisor's office projected onto the adjacent wall, displaying data gathered from the state, "which is the only factual matter that we have, I would vote that we not require masks for everyone in the district, with the exception of buses."

I looked up at the projector. On the screen were numbers of coronavirus cases from the Iowa Department of Public Health. Each week Matt and others at the county supervisors' office carefully collected data from the state to share with the community. When I communicated with Matt about the data a few days before the school board working group meeting, he mentioned that the state kept adding coronavirus case numbers to May and June, so he was trying to fix the dataset. They published a tightly organized and easily understandable graph on the Lakes Regional Healthcare Facebook page weekly.

Sharon went on to question how close kids could sit together on buses and questioned who and how they would monitor it. She stated with some uncertainty: "I would also like to say that a week from now I would like the chance to change my mind because that could change and I think we need to have a very flexible system at school."

Sharon paused and looked around the room and blurted, "Spreadsheets! I love spreadsheets! I'll hook you up!" Zach and I looked at each other, unsure where she was going. "So, we are tracking cases. I mean just being more intentional about all of it. So, that we have planned out because that has been my biggest frustration since March. We have taken away all of these opportunities from kids. Track, you name it: tennis, half the softball season, prom, dance recitals. I tell you, I can give you a longer list."

She was getting energized. "And we didn't even have any [cases]." Sharon paused and looked down at her notes,

"I mean, we had one case, and it wasn't until a month ago really, and who knows, nobody knows if we did the right thing. And we don't know what the right thing is moving forward. And I refuse to take away people's choice without solid data! I would hate to take away those choices from the kids and that is my vote today."

I sat there soaking in the differences of opinion and thought about who Sharon was speaking to. I remembered a comment from a mother I had spoken to who was conflicted about masks, and wondered if this was the large swatch of parents she was representing. The mother said, "There is [a lot of fear]. And think about it. What happens when you've got an eight-year-old with the flu? And then they get a cold and they have a runny nose but they have a mask on so their mask gets dirty. What are you gonna do? Are you gonna change out their mask six times a day because kids get snotty noses? I just don't think they're ready for this. And then like a lady asked the other day like, what happens when a teacher gets sick?"

She went on to explain, "Okay so my oldest daughter's gonna be in [high school at Spirit Lake]. And right now, they're set to go back to school. Like we are in full swing registration like we are going back. And we got her class schedule and she still sees eight teachers per day and somebody asked, 'what happens when a teacher says I'm positive for COVID?' [. . .] Like is it just gonna be a constant disruption?"

Later the mother elaborated on her concerns about masking. "In my opinion, healthy people should not have to wear a mask. I think it's causing other problems."

"Like what problems?" I asked.

"Like health problems, like lung problems. Say that you work at McDonald's and you're a healthy eighteen-year-old girl that's never had lung problems in her life. And she goes to McDonald's and she works an eight- or nine-hour shift and she wears a mask the whole day. After eight to nine hours, she takes the mask off. Well, that's eight, nine hours of breathing in your own CO_2! [. . .] And I think that when people do that, there's gonna be so many other lung problems and pulmonary problems that come from wearing a mask. Because people are gonna work and over work and over exert. And people are gonna have hypertension and heart attacks." She went on to explain, "it's just gonna be a matter of time and it's all gonna roll into one thing and they're gonna be like 'Well it's one of those things. If we lost five hundred for the greater good, then I guess it was really worth it.' And it's not."

Her fear resonated with a large part of the community (even though these fears of carbon dioxide causing harm from masks were refuted).[1] What will masks do to our kids? I thought the conflation of risk—which Sharon also emphasized—was compromising what the greater good meant. Some parents believed it would be wrong to inflict pain upon children by mandating children to wear a mask; they perceived it could cause health problems. Others believed masks should be voluntary because mandating masks jeopardized their freedoms and threatened to keep their kids home from school if masks were mandated. Was the greater good about politics or health?

How cases would be tracked was also a big point of contention. Angela, the STEM coordinator who had become the district COVID administrator, continued explaining contact tracing at the working group meeting. She had put a great deal of energy into thinking through how to figure out who was exposed to coronavirus and by whom. She explained that she and the nurse, Katie, had developed "a plan going forward of using spreadsheets, Google forms, tracking information, getting [a tech] to help us with additional coding so that we know the day that [the person] tested positive. The day they come back we have ideas for a form for parents to fill out or call in daily with issues, because that is good for the other families. But we are not going to see their kid when they are quarantined, we are not going to see their kid when they are at home. [. . .] But we do have control over if a kid is quarantined and has to be home for a few days we do know that and we can track that and we will track that."

The nurse followed up, "It is a script for everybody answering at home. It is just a basic script and everybody answering the phone just has to circle."

Sharon interjected, somewhat facetiously, "there have been so many good things that come out of this. I mean, we have had sixty kids in one day gone from the elementary school because of flu or strep throat. But I had the head of the Okoboji [school board], the president, call me and say, 'Half of our middle school has gone. Has half your middle school gone? What is going on?' I'm like, 'I don't know. Over 50 percent of the middle school was gone.' So this is a new normal. Might be a good thing, but this is not anything new. Do you know what I'm saying to a certain extent?"

Kristin responded, "The gravity of COVID is greater than influenza or any other."

Sharon agreed, "Because we just don't have a vaccine or whatever?"

"Yeah," Shane agreed.

Kristin stated, "You know how I feel about masks, but what about when social distancing cannot be maintained, for hallways. How is that . . ."

Sharon jumped in again, "I thought we had every fifteen minutes?" By now Zach's knee was bouncing and he was talking under his breath, which he now says he regrets. The CDC had recommended that people not spend more than fifteen minutes inside together in close quarters and somehow this had morphed into an unmovable policy for how students would move throughout the school day. Zach's colleagues had spent a frustrating meeting with the administration and it was clear that the school board was setting the six feet in proximity for fifteen minutes guidelines in stone. It was becoming the Golden Rule.

They went on to discuss school lunches—should kids be able to leave campus? Will music practice continue? How do they do this safely? The superintendent complained that the public health department shut down the marching band's practice just hours before the meeting because no one was following any social distancing rules. Eventually they returned to issues of space, the major discussion point that most people agreed upon: make plenty of space for students to spread out, and they can sing, play an instrument, or kick a ball. The high school principal said, "I think the issue is going to be getting them to hang out. They will find every nook and cranny. But that is our job, to change all of the hang out areas. There are going to be new rules put up."

The superintendent summarized, "We are all on the same page. We are doing more to explore additional space right now. Our plan is to try as hard as we possibly can to have everyone, if possible, six feet apart. The main core learning time, we understand there is going to be time for the hallways and passing, and transitions and buses and lunch room. Other than the core learning time, we are going to really look at that. So, we are not stopping unless somebody tells us different like six and a half feet—that is why we put the six feet into place unless it changes. I think six feet is good. And we are doing the fifteen-minute thing is good. We are going to rotate the kids through a little faster than normal. So, we are trying to pay attention to that and make sure we are doing it, I don't think we can stop the bus every fourteen minutes and rotate."[2] Everything felt very final. Like the administration would move kids through the school—packed together in buses, hallways, and music class—but only for fifteen minutes, without masks.

I could not stop thinking about the security and finality they associated with these six feet and fifteen minute designations. *Viruses don't follow time, and they can move beyond six feet. You cannot see them.*

Sharon said, soft on the side, "I'm disappointed contact tracing has to happen if you are wearing a mask."

"If you are wearing a mask, it goes back to six feet, fifteen minutes," the superintendent stated, demonstrating that this golden rule was solidified in his mind.

"It helps prevent diseases!" Zach stated from the observation area. He was increasingly frustrated that, besides Kristin, there were no scientists permitted to speak. The school board members were leaning toward requiring no masks at all. There were at least ten health professionals watching, and not one was invited to engage with the school board working group in this open session for the community.

ENDORSING CAUTION

At the end of the working session, Zach put his hand up, and then down. He was not invited to speak, and did not want to interfere. He put his hand up, and then down again. I whispered, "Just stand up, Zach! They might not see you!" Zach asked to speak three or four times before the superintendent acknowledged him. Principals sitting near us were literally waving their hands to get the superintendent's attention.

As the chair of the board of health, he was compelled to share his perspective in a decision he thought about every day. As a parent and physician, he felt masking was critical. But Zach also realized that people on the school board considered him, as Dr. Fauci said the Trump administration viewed him, as "the skunk at the picnic."[3]

"I'm Zach. I'm the chair of the board of health. Thank you for letting me speak, and I apologize for interrupting. I think looking at all of this as 'masks are not going to protect me' is misguided. I'm wearing a mask really to protect you guys. I'm wearing a medical mask because I have one and that protects me from all of these people sitting here with no masks on in this small enclosed space. But it is helping everybody else so they are not exposed to me." He was speaking quickly, nervous but calm.

"The fifteen minutes and six feet [rule] is all about a level of risk. I could be sitting six feet away from someone and be terribly infected and cough on someone for two seconds. And really, if enough particles come out of my mouth and go into their lungs, they can get it. So the six feet is not magic. I mean, more is better. Six feet is the lesser recommendation. If you can't be outside of six feet, then ideally you are wearing a mask. And there is nothing magic about fifteen minutes either! And if the [students] are rotating every fourteen minutes, that means that more people are going to get exposed. It is about being in smaller groups and trying to keep those interactions smaller and keeping those groups smaller."

"I'm thinking about this every day all day," Zach continued. "I know that I've contacted all of you. And I appreciate that this is an untenable situation for you guys to be in, especially given the lack of a higher level of guidance [from the state]. The information on how contact tracing is going to happen hasn't even come out from the state. And so, they are giving you their best answers now because again [the public health personnel] haven't gotten the information. It would have been better had they been given the information about what they are responsible for and when it is appropriate to contact your local health department. When the public health department hasn't been informed of what that responsibility is, it is really challenging."

Zach spoke on, quickly but assertively, as the school board members stared, seemingly dismissively. "We would all love to have more answers but really the best answer is be as careful as possible. And so I would love to see masks not because I want to force against anybody's rights, but because my rights are being taken away if you are sick and not wearing one around me. In all reality, my right to health and safety is being taken away. I agree and I'm no legal person by any means, but you know we require shirts, we require pants, we require a level of conduct. And so if it is part of the dress code, especially if there are opt-outs, whether it is for a doctor or an IEP [individualized education plan] or something along those lines. We do that for immunizations. I'll stop talking but thank you for letting me comment. Thank you."

The working session ended, and everyone left. Zach had to speak to colleagues and other local officials so I slid out the door. I chatted with a family friend who was a health provider and parent. She was exasperated by the meeting. How could they be so flippant about masks? It's such a small thing—a piece of cloth you wrap around your face. As we chatted—in masks—one school board member scurried out the door, maskless. She clearly did not want to engage. She said over her shoulder, "I'm going to pray real hard!," indicating that this was a huge decision—one that she never wanted to have to face. The school board members had exactly one week left to think about how they would vote on the final public health provisions for the upcoming school year. For many people, the immensely political and contested environment was not something they would have anticipated when running for the board.

CHAPTER 13

SATURDAY

AS I MULLED over the discussion and division from the school board working session, I was writing a short piece about what I had observed in Okoboji over the summer. I started working on the piece at the peak of the June outbreak—first submitting versions to regional papers including the *Des Moines Register* and the *Sioux City Journal.* These regional news outlets didn't bite so I reached out to Dan Byman, a colleague at Georgetown and fellow Midwesterner, for some advice. My colleague provided feedback on the piece—as writing for the public is quite different than the academic writing I usually do. Dan also sent some introductory emails for me to connect with science editors at national news outlets. It was through these networks that the piece landed at *Vox.*

It just so happened that my final edits were due to the editor at *Vox* the day after the school board meeting. The article was titled "How an Iowa Summer Resort Region Became a Covid-19 Hot Spot: A Medical Anthropologist on Why the Coronavirus Response Is So Controversial in Her Hometown." I discussed how the community fractured around decisions to mask or unmask, and how some people ditched masks for political reasons and others did it for economic ones.[1] I wrote, "For instance, if you wear a mask around here, it reflects defiance against President Trump. When masks became this sort of political statement, most people described feeling deeply hurt—simply due to the divergent views that were (or weren't) now spread across their faces."

My head was spinning as I edited the piece and I decided to use my pen to make a point as the school year inched closer. I added an additional critique about school decisions, trying to shine a light on the seriousness of the upcoming school board decision and the conflicting Midwestern values that emerged. I wrote, "This division recently came to a head in a heated open school board meeting on August 3 about reopening schools. Many board members invoked 'freedom' and 'individual choice' in their comments on masking at schools." I also suggested that "these conflicts are being fostered by a lack of local political support for public health measures, which reflects the greater coronavirus tragedy in the American Midwest. The superintendent of the school district, for example, plans to open schools with few safety measures in place, despite the local public health leaders providing opposing advice."

I first drafted the piece when cases were at their peak, and described how despite being a hotspot, many called coronavirus a hoax or pushed on to enjoy a normal summer. I wrote about the common expression from June, explaining how people said, "Everyone has COVID!" I also shared how other people worried "nobody will take it seriously until someone prominent in the community dies." At that point, six people had died, including some who were well known, and many people explained away their deaths by age, body size, and pre-existing health conditions.

I also described how Richard Ashby, who was visiting his family in Milford, was harassed at a gas station over the July Fourth weekend. Lori Eich, my oldest friend, who helped with this project, texted me a screenshot of his post and I followed up with him. Richard posted onto social media:

> My boyfriend and I just got harassed for wearing masks walking into a convenience store by a group of about six guys who were probably between 18 and 20. As we walked by one of the guys yelled, "Corona virus isn't real." We told them "Yeah, we're from Texas, we know people who have died." This quickly escalated into a barrage of strange insults and some of the guys walking up to us like they were ready to throw down. We told them to calm down, wash their hands and wear a mask. When we exited the store they continued with their insults, one of them walking towards us and then away like he was ready to fight. As we walked into the street a guy who had been parked at the store pulled up to us and told us he admired our resolve. We just shrugged. "We don't know what that was."[2]

Despite some of these thoughtless acts, many people were deeply committed to each other. I wrote how "I spoke to a manager at Menards, a regional home improvement chain, who said they have been required to wear masks since March. When the staff first was required to wear masks, she made extras for her coworkers who had fewer means. She said it wasn't a big deal and wants to keep herself, family, and community safe. Although, she notes, they are occasionally harassed by customers."

I concluded with a message to the community: "Only by understanding one another and rebuilding trust in our institutions, science, and each other can we come out of this crisis stronger."

RESPONSE

The piece came out the morning of August 8, when there was a Trump boat parade organized on West Lake Okoboji. The boat parade was hosted by John Wills as well as other local political activists (who I found out later also attended the rally that occurred right before the insurrection attempt in Washington, DC, on January 6, 2021). The parade involved people gathering in boats adorned with flags, signs, and rallying calls to express support for the president in a heated election year. Some boats had flags with mixed messages, which complicated the political and cultural dynamics at play in their political movement (e.g., Confederate flags, Trump 2020 flags, and one that said "Jesus is my Savior, Trump is my President"—furthering the messianic role many perceived Trump fulfilled).

They congregated in front of Arnolds Park Amusement Park and puttered slowly around the perimeter of the lake, taking around an hour to complete the loop, with

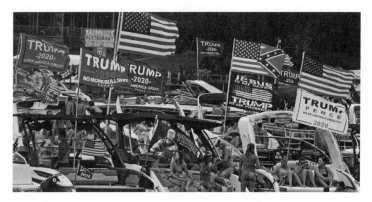

FIGURE 13.1. Flags at the Trump boat parade. Courtesy of David Thoreson.

one boat following the other. Campus Radio said that an eyewitness observed "hundreds" of boats at the political rally.[3] I saw around fifty.

I started getting texts early in the morning after the article was released. Usually when I publish something—an academic journal article, a commentary, or a book—only about a handful of people take notice. This was different.

My mom was the first to text me. She was reading it in bed. At first, I thought it might be another piece of writing that only my mom reads.

But then my friends from childhood started texting me. They'd found it! How fun!

By late morning my friends from other parts of my life found it and sent varying messages from "Stay safe!" to "These pictures are crazy! Are these from this summer?" The pictures had been taken by my friend David Thoreson only a few weeks prior, on July Fourth. David also happens to be an adventure photographer who is well known throughout the Iowa Great Lakes Region for his beautiful photos of crashing waves, racing sailboats, and August sunsets.

When the article was posted on Facebook, there were a variety of replies. One man said, "I've had lots of friends from around the globe sending me this. Nice to see it's gaining some traction." Another woman said, "Great article and so sorry this is happening in such an idyllic spot." A classmate, who had moved away only recently, posted, "The Iowa Great Lakes can no longer pride themselves on being 'community minded' given their behavior and lack of empathy for mankind over the past 4 months."

Some people wanted more nuance to the article. A man posted, "This is not political to me. My main point was to wish the author would have posted recovery rates instead of making people in her hometown look like a bunch of irresponsible hicks. That I truly believe was her point. It was a jab at us who still live here. The article was factually true, but misleading at the same time." This one made me scratch my head—*my family lives in Okoboji!*

A woman responded to him: "If the rates are low in Dickinson County, it's because of those people who follow the advice of scientists and medical professionals; to stay home, wear masks when they have to be out, practice social distancing, avoid bars, restaurants, church services, etc." I nodded my head as I read this; I had found this dichotomy throughout the summer where most locals were being cautious while some vocal and visible ones were not.

He responded, "The sheep wear masks in Walmart. That is basically the only place. We are doing just fine. Me? I have never and will never put a mask on. Please stay in your own lane in Lakefield. Stay home."

Others were openly aggressive to me. A woman I had reached out to about an interview, but from whom I had never received a response, sent me a private Facebook message. She was a friend of a friend who a couple people had suggested I speak to because she was very vocal about anti-masking. She sent three messages in succession at 6:38 p.m.

"I am so glad I never talked to you. You are the problem not the solution! I hope you enjoyed the Trump Boat Parade today! Americans enjoying their freedoms at the Iowa Great Lakes! Shame on you for writing such a racist article about your home! I never want to know you!"

Moments later, this followed:

"Obviously you are NOT a healthcare provider & you like to stir the pot! Stay in Washington you belong there! You want to say Christians & White people are racist your article is racist! Obviously your parents failed you!"

And a final blow, which made me chuckle: "Professors are the worst! Bleeding Liberals!"

It wasn't the first hate mail I'd received but it certainly didn't feel good. She sent it off around cocktail hour on a Saturday, so maybe she had been drinking. Yet I was curious about why she thought the article was racist and why it made her so angry that she would send me a personal message filled with so much vitriol.

Perhaps more difficult was that I hurt the feelings of someone I consider a friend because I quoted something she shared with me during an interview (she could not have known, but in fact multiple people communicated the same message to me).

In response to an email that I had sent out to all study participants with a link to the article, most replied with brief messages like, "Wonderful!" "Terrific!" and "Thanks for sharing! How interesting!" Others never responded but I saw them post messages on Facebook like, "Everyone just be kind to each other."

One interview participant shared three immediate responses:

"I'm surprised at the mask-wearing-as-political-statement wrinkle.

"The hotspot numbers are diluted as tourists head back home.

"David's photos—sadly—do more to illustrate the problem for me than mere words."

We went back and forth about different observations he had about the article. Then, his final email made my eyes bulge as it was accompanied with a photo of the Barefoot Bar chock full of densely packed-together patrons watching a performance on stage. He said, "I take this seriously— my neighbor, an ER nurse, went to Elmhurst Memorial [to work] for 13 weeks. She came back [to the Iowa Great Lakes] and contracted COVID-19 and was hospitalized for 2 weeks. She's home now, but very weak. So . . . When the Barefoot Bar hosted the very popular Johnny Holm Band, I went on to their webcam. Just before showtime, I saw Butch and Debbie meet up with Johnny. They elbow-bumped . . . and then Butch gave Johnny a big hug. (So what was the play-it-safe elbow bump about?). Here's another reason why I worry about events that attract tourists and locals. The next week should be interesting to watch. I title this photo 'What Could Possibly Go Wrong?'"

The last email was from a restaurant owner who had battled COVID risks all summer. The comment made me look two days into the future when the next school board meeting was scheduled: "Great article and accurate comments. It will really be interesting to see how the school part plays out. Many teachers I've talked to want required masking. My thinking is these schools and boards aren't 'in it' yet. Once they are truly faced with the decision of closing due to a few positives they may make different decisions."

I thought about this final comment throughout the next day and into Monday. Hours later the school board was planning to vote on masking in schools. What would they choose?

CHAPTER 14

GLITCH

THE FINAL WORKING group meeting on school policies
was two days later, again on Monday. This time we met
in a large room in the media center at the high school. It
was moved to this large space at the last minute, and we
had trouble figuring out where we should go. Every school
board member was sitting six feet away from others. The
chairs for spectators were spaced apart. On one side of
the room were people who were largely unmasked. On the
other side of the room were people who were masked. I
arrived with my sister, Kate, and her husband, Zach, who
said they wanted to sit apart from me. (I agreed, happy to
take the heat for causing a stink in national media about
this particular meeting.) I saw an old friend who rode
the bus with me throughout our childhoods. I waved; she
looked away.

Living in a small town causes a lot of social pressure,
and Kate and Zach were worried about the social fallout
of my article. They also had prepared statements for the
end of the meeting. I took an empty chair in the front so
I could record the meeting.

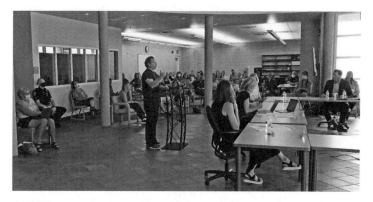

FIGURE 14.1. School board meeting. Courtesy of David Thoreson.

The meeting was relatively quick. Each board member shared their statements: very brief and to the point. They had agreed that they would require masking in hallways, on buses, when people were in close proximity. Kristin suggested they mandate masking for both the high school and middle school students. The others agreed that students would be required to put on a mask in the hallways, buses, and whenever people could not keep six feet apart (like when students got up to go to the bathroom in class).[1]

The public forum was quick but pointed. One woman was worried because her child was living with a disability and could not handle a mask. Another woman home-schooled her children but, as a well-known anti-vaxxer evangelist, wanted to argue that building immunity was key and that masks were uncalled for. Kate spoke about why masking was important for keeping her children and the community safe. Zach gave a similar short speech as well.

The public forum ended with a physician in Zach's practice contradicting him, suggesting that masks didn't matter at all. Science was conflicted, he said, "There is not any evidence out there right now that strongly suggests that masks are going to prevent the transmission. Now you are going to have articles on this side, articles on that side; they are going back and forth. It is—that argument is not going to end." He was not wearing a mask.

The five school board members voted on requiring masks in hallways, buses, bathrooms—any time students were in close proximity. Even though students could remove their masks when they sat at their desks—spaced six feet apart—the relative mask mandate was much more stringent than what had been discussed the week before in the school board working group.

Each one of the five school board members voted for the mask mandate.

We were shocked but excited.

After the meeting, Zach was thrilled. He said, "I think the article may have influenced the vote. I don't think they would have required masking without the social pressure." I smiled, thinking, Maybe academics can be helpful in the public health effort, after all?

But I was also disheartened. At the end of the day, it seemed that only one thing made the school board take public health seriously when no federal or state mandates were in place: shame.

DATA

On the following Monday morning, I read the headline "'Horrifying' Data Glitch Skews Key Iowa Coronavirus

Metrics." I shook my head and thought, What in the world? I took a slug of coffee and thought back to Sharon's primary reasoning for not requiring masks: the state's data was "the only factual matter that we have." Based on that data, she said, "I would vote that we not require masks for everyone in the district." I could not help but think that this point fractured when news broke that the state data was incomplete. There was a data "glitch."

Ryan Foley of the Associated Press reported the data error in the governor's office. Apparently, the state had been underrepresenting the number of new confirmed cases and the severity of the current outbreak. Foley wrote, "The glitch means the Iowa Department of Public Health has inadvertently been reporting fewer new infections and a smaller percentage of daily positive tests than is truly the case, according to Dana Jones, an Iowa City nurse practitioner who uncovered the problem. It's particularly significant because school districts are relying on state data to determine whether they will offer in-person instruction when school resumes in the coming days and weeks."[2] This "data glitch" occurred just as school boards across the state of Iowa, including Spirit Lake, were deliberating about whether or not to require masks as they sent thousands of students back to school.

Ryan Foley wrote again two days later, "An aggressive push by Iowa's pro-Trump governor to reopen schools amid a worsening coronavirus outbreak has descended into chaos, with some districts and teachers rebelling and experts calling the scientific benchmarks used by the state arbitrary and unsafe."[3] He attributed this obfuscation of cases by the governor's office a ploy to support President Trump's agenda, to trick school boards into thinking the coronavirus pandemic was getting better. This may have been related to Trump's words (or intent) in July when he had warned schools against going virtual: "We would like to see schools open. We want to see the economy open. I would like to see the schools open—open 100%. And we'll do it safely; we'll do it carefully."[4]

I reached out to other state legislators to get some perspective on the purported data glitch. A Democratic state legislator from southern Iowa was frank with me about the numbers. He explained, "The state of Iowa's not being transparent with testing. The glitches are deceptive. [. . .] If an individual was tested a second and subsequent time, they're still only going to count that as one test. So, the state of Iowa was back-dating all these current tests to the date that a person was first tested, which created this deception that the rate was higher back then than it was today. And they knowingly did that, which was terrible."

The data errors were confirmed by an Iowa Department of Public Health official who said "a system-generated date on which test results were reported to the state stayed the same when an individual later tested positive."[5] Governor Kim Reynolds explained, "We're continuing to work with an antiquated system. There continue to be issues with trying to take a system that was never designed to deal with the amount of data that we're feeding through it."[6] Although state officials knew of the glitch in late July, and the governor said she was not aware of the glitch until a week before the story broke (the day of the Spirit Lake school board vote), misleading data appeared to have been knowingly released to the public for weeks.[7] Many people remained skeptical that the data had been fixed.[8]

CHAPTER 15

FOMO

I LEFT OKOBOJI on August 15, the day after my sister's birthday. At the end of each summer, I feel a deep sadness in the pit of my stomach, combined with excitement for the year to come. Leaving has become ever more difficult since my sister moved back to Okoboji. I see my kids do the same jumps and wiggles into the lake as I did when I was young. The pull of my family and the lake feels stronger each year, generations deep.

When my second grader prepared for a year of virtual schooling, I wondered if we should have stayed in Okoboji. My niece and nephew returned to school with their classmates on August 24. Parents were delighted to get their kids out of the house, but many were nervous. On Facebook, people posted back-to-school pictures, with most of the kids in masks. My sister said my nephew asked to go to school earlier and earlier each day so he could have extra time to play on the playground with his friends. Part of my heart broke as I thought about how isolated my daughter was, the same age, doing virtual school at home.

I continued to speak with many of my interlocutors throughout the school year, touching base at random times, when I heard about curious gossip or news. In October, I reconnected with Mary, the teacher I spoke to in July who described how the pandemic put her on a corona-coaster, to see how the school year was going.

Mary said, "Things have I think gone smashing here, compared to what we thought it might look like." I thought skeptically about this comment for a minute because the amount of community transmission of coronavirus had increased steadily since the schools had opened.

"We feel like we went about it the right way," Mary continued. "I can see in my class, and right now it's ginormous, but we're definitely social distancing. And the kids wear their masks at least where we as a school district had required masks in the hallways. At least in the beginning, we had one kid who maybe was trying to fight that. Like start a petition, you know, and was putting negative things on Instagram or whatever. But it died down pretty quick. Even kids—where families that didn't love the mask idea—when you talk with them, they're like, it's just not worth it. I want to keep playing football and I literally have to wear a mask like fourteen minutes a day."

Mary explained her own risk perspective, too. "I was talking to a senior and they can sit in their desks and take their masks down as long as they are six feet apart. They can have them off. The one thing as a teacher that's been hard is that I feel like I'm not with them for very long. But when I would definitely get right up in their business, you don't now. I mean, it's hard not to. It's hard not to just bend right down to them and they don't have their masks on. I have mine on, but I lean right down and teach. Right? So this is one thing that has been a bit stressful. A couple teachers did try to sell to the kids to mask when they come near them, or whatever. I guess I've tried to sort of work through it like I move away pretty quick. I don't know, it's hard."

Mary went on to explain that students were concerned about coronavirus because they had FOMO: *fear of missing out*. FOMO was mostly associated with the process of contact tracing, which was stressful for students because it meant that, if a student was in proximity to someone who was COVID-positive, then they would be required to quarantine for two weeks. This included not only attending school virtually but also missing out on school-related activities for that two-week period.

She said, "The whole cheerleading squad had to quarantine after they did contact tracing. At the time, for the Department of Public Health, it didn't matter if you had masks on. So even the kids that had masks on, and were within six feet for fifteen minutes, had to quarantine. And so that came back to bite us a little bit."

Mary felt that masking mandates when students were close to each other mattered, suggesting that the school board made the right decision to require some masking.

But some people kept trying to bend the rules. A mom friend told me, "Apparently the high school's getting a lot of COVID cases. Two coaches are out, and I just heard that there's a couple kids, at least a couple on the JV football team. One kid tested positive and then they're doing contact tracing and so a bunch of kids are on quarantine. The whole cheerleading squad is out of high school. Apparently, there's like eight kids on the high school varsity football team that have lost their sense of taste and have one or two other symptoms. But they are not telling anyone because the homecoming game is this Friday and they don't wanna knock out the whole team." I had heard these rumors from others, too.

At Sibley, a neighboring school, "a number of their football team members got COVID and they knocked out fifty kids in the whole school." School officials were forced to cancel homecoming as a result.[1] "So there's definitely a feeling that you could knock out your whole team if you're honest and transparent about it. And with homecoming, there's not a lot of motivation to be transparent because you might not get to play and your team might be out from quarantine and contact tracing."

The parent went on to explain more about the Sibley student, "who knocked out the whole football team. He tested positive and was open about it and then stayed home. But a lot of people got coronavirus and I guess he was getting death threats."

I gasped. "Oh my God! So, he stayed home and then all the kids around him had to stay home? And then . . ."

"Yeah, because football is such a big deal and he was honest and caused everyone else to stay home because that's the responsible thing to do." She shook her head. "Without someone leaving a moral for like—let's be kind to each other and let's do what's right and that this is just like a crappy time in history where we all have to just follow the guidelines and we're doing it to keep everyone safe—without someone saying that message, people are just being mad about it. And it's inconvenient and maybe a hoax or something. I mean, I think that was stressful for teachers and parents that that happened not too far from here."

While it may or may not have been true that athletes were covering up symptoms, the fact is that the school year went relatively well, despite a lack of transparency. Students attended class and had a relatively normal school year. (At least, *normal* compared to children around the country attending school virtually.) Even while many students and teachers spent time in quarantine for positive test results or potential exposures, school continued without any official break or prolonged disruption.

Yet, at the same time, community transmission skyrocketed when school started. In a letter dated November 16, 2020, the Dickinson County Board of Health cited "a significant rise in hospitalizations over the last month" associated with COVID-19.[2] They asked the Dickinson County Board of Supervisors—the governing body most locals considered responsible for managing the outbreak, and who was tracking it closely—to consider a proclamation to use masks county wide. At the same time, the board of health (again) asked Governor Reynolds to consider a masking mandate at the state level.

One county supervisor, Kim Wermerson, said publicly at a meeting about masking in November, "For me, the bottom line is we're in crisis." The supervisor indicated that they had been in discussion with several medical professionals. "They're saying they need help. I think we have to react to that. I don't think we as supervisors have the authority to out-mandate the governor. However, I am in favor of us passing some sort of (proclamation) saying we are definitely in favor of masks being worn."[3]

The CEO of the hospital supported Zach and the other members of Dickinson County Public Health, stating, "I think as that spread has occurred and has impacted the hospital in a more significant way. I have really changed my thinking about that. Quite honestly—whichever studies you believe at this point—if universal masking was 10 percent effective and kept an additional hospital bed open, that minor inconvenience, in my mind, is worth it." [4]

The mandate failed, although the board of supervisors supported the governor's proclamation from November 16.[5] Seth Boyes of the *Dickinson County News* noted that "Supervisor Tim Fairchild said the most common point of contention he's heard regarding mask use is the potential encroachment on individual freedom."[6]

The next week my Facebook feed filled with photos of friends celebrating Friendsgiving in the Iowa Great Lakes region. Others posted photos of arriving at warm beaches for quick holidays away from the chilly November Iowa weather. One school board member posted photos of her family in Florida, in front of an ice cream store, grinning without masks. Others posted normal photos of gatherings like it was any other year. Perhaps I noticed these photos this year because I had not seen my family since August. I had stayed in Iowa just long enough to celebrate my sister's birthday. Usually my family then comes to me for the Thanksgiving holiday. We wake up early and run the Turkey

Trot around the capital before we hustle home to turn on the oven for the turkey. But this year their chairs were empty.

After the Christmas holiday season came and went, Okoboji's big winter festival weekend was fast approaching: the University of Okoboji Winter Games. I thought for a moment that the Winter Games would be cancelled, but then my sister mentioned on the phone one day how disappointed she was to miss the Chili Cookoff. They cancelled the indoor events: the Chili Cookoff, Chocolate Classic, and Cribbage Tournament. Outdoor events were still scheduled, but the chamber encouraged people to wear masks and practice social distancing for the 10K race, polar plunge, ice hockey competition, ice fishing, and fireworks.[7] Kate and Zach said the socially distanced s'mores outside Boathouse Apparel were sticky and delicious, and the polar plunge looked especially cold as people cannonballed into a hole in the frozen lake. I saw on Facebook how many people still gathered indoors unmasked to celebrate the one weekend of revelry tourists came into town to share amid the winter months.

Governor Reynolds rolled back public health restrictions a week after Winter Games and just days before Super Bowl Sunday. By March and April, the Iowa Great Lakes saw a spike in cases that rivaled that of the previous June.[8] This peak was larger than the greatest peak in November and December, with thirty- and forty-somethings filling hospital beds. Yet the community gave a collective yawn.

By mid-May, around 2,700 people had tested positive for COVID-19—around 16 percent of the residents of Dickinson County. Forty-four people had died.[9]

But things improved once vaccines arrived because many people were eager to get them. By May 18, 2021, 80 percent of Dickinson County residents over sixty-five years of age were fully vaccinated, as were 55 percent of those eighteen years and older.[10] Many families who had been exceedingly careful throughout the pandemic began to resume their pre-pandemic lives.

But public health urged people to be cautious, while many community members felt life was returning to normal. The county supervisors voted on April 27 to remove a mask mandate that was still in place at the courthouse. The next day the Spirit Lake school board "lifted mask requirements." This was three days before prom.[11]

Spirit Lake's graduation was held on May 16 in the high school gymnasium. A couple graduates wore masks but I'm unsure how many in the crowd wore masks. Okoboji High School graduation was a week later. They celebrated Brian Downing—the principal at Okoboji High School who had been shamed for promoting masks—who was named Iowa's High School Principal of the Year.[12]

As summer approached and the restrictions were eased, pre-pandemic life resumed. The 100 days of summer were afoot. For many, the pandemic was over.

EPILOGUE

WRITING A BOOK about a pandemic in the middle of a pandemic seems ridiculous. But there is something to learn about these first days when people resisted even the belief that the pandemic was real in Okoboji, while the affliction circumnavigated the globe. America's use of personal responsibility as a national or state strategy amid the first year of the pandemic was a complete failure. This was not because people failed to care for each other—in many situations, people used logics of care to think about and care for those most vulnerable in their lives. But this strategy extended to businesses and conflated local businesses with people, as America is prone to do. When businesses were not mandated to follow public health guidelines, many put profit before people. They undermined the efforts of local public health departments, exemplifying how an uncoordinated response breaks down and destabilizes the arduous work of public health. Documenting the breakdown of the American response, and how different it was compared to the rest of the world, matters. In public health and medicine, it is important to write about *what did not work* as much as to write about *what did*.

It is late spring of 2021 as I struggle to write this, an epilogue about an ongoing pandemic. Vaccines are spreading throughout the United States, at least among those who can and will receive them. My parents were vaccinated in early January, as was Zach. My husband was vaccinated in February because he was teaching in person each week at Johns Hopkins University. My cousin Hannah found me a vaccine appointment at a Walgreens while scrolling for appointments in the middle of the night once professors became eligible in March; it is unfathomable to me how people who do not know my cousin Hannah ever found a vaccine appointment then. However, a month later, adults could drop into any pharmacy for a COVID vaccine when they were picking up shampoo. Access to life-saving technology was truly a testament to the amazing speed with which vaccines were developed; but at the same time, who had access to those vaccines was deeply uneven. It remains unclear when people in other countries, even those that responded quicker and better than the United States, will have them.

In March I spoke with a faculty member from a university in Kigali, Rwanda. When she asked what I was up to, I mentioned this book. She said, "Well, we've done a great job here. The government shut everything down and has tightly controlled the spread. It's been incredible to see people come together like this."[1] Indeed, many African countries like Rwanda responded swiftly and more confidently than wealthier countries like the United States in preventing the spread of SARS-CoV-2, leading to many fewer casualties.² Although global health leaders from the United States and Europe offered their guidance on policy or prevention early in the pandemic, many countries, like Rwanda, did not need their input. These conversations about who should lead and why could not be more vital than at this moment. There is so much at stake in the leadership of global health policy, where people are (re)thinking where knowledge and power sit, recognizing whose voices matter, why, and where.

My experience in my hometown solidified a question that I constantly grapple with: What does it mean to do meaningful work globally when things are such a mess locally? When I was studying at Davidson College, I volunteered at local health clinics in North Carolina and Iowa, mostly to learn and observe. I filed papers, cleaned rooms, and set up spaces for snacks or waiting areas. Later, I observed the deeper systemic challenges facing the public healthcare system over the several years I worked at the old Cook County Hospital in Chicago. Through these experiences I realized how broken and fragmented the American healthcare system is. I also realized how critical politics and policies were for framing people's health; it is not only access to medical care that drives good health. Social, economic, ecological, and political conditions drive why and how people get infected or afflicted, and how people perceive and experience that affliction ultimately shapes people's health.

In an interview with her alma mater, Rebecca Katz reflected on the pandemic. "The biggest failure of our community might have been the failure of imagination," she explained. "We all intellectually knew that a pandemic was a possibility. We also knew exactly where the fault lines were. Maybe the important lesson is that we need to yell louder and make sure that we are collectively heard when we talk about the importance of preparedness."[3] In essence, Rebecca emphasized, in her careful and thoughtful way, that scientific expertise was sidelined and public health authorities were muffled.

Political actions by the Trump administration did not reflect recommendations from the public health and medical communities. Ignoring scientific expertise crippled America's ability to control the pandemic, resulting in more death and devastation than anywhere else in the world (although as I edit these pages, COVID-19 has surged in India and Brazil, transforming many places into humanitarian emergencies). Political leadership in the United States by some state governors certainly did contribute to lower rates of death, such as in Minnesota, where the governor took swift and aggressive measures to shut down the state. The Minnesota-Iowa border sits just twenty miles from Okoboji. We saw over and over again how states that opened up too early, or shut down too late, experienced more virus and deaths than places that enforced public health measures early and often. We know that coordinated leadership matters.

The power of leadership in mitigating the rippling effect of COVID-19 could not be more apparent than in New Zealand. New Zealand's prime minister Jacinda Ardern took public health data seriously, closed down the island to outside travel, and controlled the spread through compassionate leadership. Rachel Blacher, a public health classmate of mine who describes herself as a former CDC staffer and expat living in New Zealand, explained the prime minister's response best for *Atlanta* magazine. "The Prime Minister made the right decision to 'go hard, go early' by imposing a four-week lockdown on March 25, when there were still very few cases in the country, with an ambitious goal to eliminate transmission of the virus. Making that decision was undoubtedly hard because there were so many variables and, in the end, could have been for naught. [. . .] Prime Minister Ardern prioritized the health and well-being of her 'team of five million' and in doing so, saved lives."[4] Rachel described the effectiveness of Ardern's communication, emphasizing "empathy and compassion in the time of crisis" and "consistently included language reminding New Zealanders to be kind and take care of each other."[5]

I write about Rachel's reflection here because I read it in the midst of the Okoboji outbreak in June of 2020. The juxtaposition of leadership between President Trump and Prime Minister Ardern was not lost on me. In fact, I felt a profound loss thinking about what a mindful leader, at a different time, with a more compassionate approach might have done. How many lives might have been saved if data more directly informed policy? How might people have treated each other with compassion, and truly cared for each other if the president, his spokespeople, and the media had spoken differently about COVID-19? How has American exceptionalism become a myth that drags us down?

The American experiment continues to test its boundaries, cohesiveness, and potential. Recognizing our multiracial democracy as something we draw on and build from is essential as we recover in the wake of an event that should shake the soul of America. It is not only the death count that should rattle us. It is how we failed to care for one another. It is how we refused to see and acknowledge the survival risks for the most vulnerable among us. These are the facts that should make us rethink whose voices matter in our collective union, and what lies at its center. With a changing climate, pandemic threats will intensify. Now is the time to rethink how we as a nation care for one another, and put "doing the right thing" for the public's health at the center of our policy as well as the fabric of our society.

ACKNOWLEDGMENTS

IT'S COMPLICATED TO write about a place you have been connected to since birth, and in which your family lives. In small towns people gossip. When I asked my sister what would happen at home, where some people might not like the book, she said probably they would gossip about something I said in seventh grade! I laughed uncomfortably. I am lucky so many of my classmates still reside in the community and many of them shared their views, experiences, and concerns with me, formally or informally, for the pages that make up this book. Reconnecting with so many old friends, mentors, teachers, and friends of friends made this project special. Thank you to everyone who responded to me, even if it was with an emoji and a frank "no!" when I asked if they wanted to talk with me about coronavirus. I appreciate you and everything you have taught me.

Reader, I must state that I wrote the book of my own accord. I am very close to my family, but they are not responsible for anything that you may not like in this book. However, let me disclose (and thank them for) the contributions they made. I observed my father, a member of the city council in Okoboji and retired physician, deliberate with others about responding to (or, in my view, mostly ignoring) the enforcement of public health recommendations. I chose deliberately not to interview him, or my mother, but we spoke informally about local government and politics throughout the summer, which is something we always do. My mother also relayed a great many helpful observations, contacts, news, and gossip. My aunt Abby Adams conducted a few interviews (after completing her ethics approval) and engaged in constant conversation with me about the project. As a retired physician and a summer resident, she stoked our ongoing dialogue about the interviews, observations, events, rumors, and everyday talk. Lori Eich, my oldest friend, also completed her ethics approval and conducted a handful of interviews; some of our conversations clarified for me what was going on, and her comments on the manuscript really made me think. My dear friend Jane Shuttleworth also fed me books about moral foundations and discussed local history, culture, and ecology in depth with me. I constantly talked about the research with my husband, Adam, too, who is a scholar of health policy—but this entwining dialogue is part of our daily life. I spoke to my sister about how the pandemic affected agriculture, and she was one of a handful of farmers I interviewed. Gentle reader, if you are upset with anything in this book, the work is mine alone.

I chose not to formally interview my brother-in-law Zachary Borus until late fall, and arranged an interview with him only when I was following up with others from the summer. I started the project in part to assist him in figuring out what was going on in Okoboji amid the June outbreak. However, we decided Zach should remain an outsider/insider. I shared my findings, questions, and considerations with him with the hope that it might assist in the public health response. We spoke constantly about his work and my observations. But only after I figured something out from an interview, did he confirm; therefore, Zach played a crucial role in confirming truth in my data by triangulating my findings from multiple convergent sources.

I am very thankful to Georgetown University for providing a semester sabbatical so that I could write this book. In all honesty, it was an overdue sabbatical because I had relinquished previous sabbaticals in exchange for a reduced teaching load while my babies were small during my pretenure years. Those were arduous years, but they were made lighter by my colleagues in the Science, Technology, and International Affairs Program and the African Studies Program in the Edmund A. Walsh School of Foreign Service. A semester-long sabbatical to write, think, and reflect on a health crisis in my hometown felt like a gift. Another gift was Diana Kim's thoughtful, generous, and kind reading of the manuscript, for which I am forever grateful.

My students, whom my late mentor Stanley O. Foster instructed me to call *learners*, walked with me in this journey via weekly meetings throughout the pandemic summer where we talked about our multiple, concurrent studies about COVID-19 in rural America as well as in Johannesburg, South Africa, where much of my ongoing research continued. Thank you to the pandemic summer research group, including my Georgetown learners Maydha Dhanuka, Natalie Kim, Syona Hariharan, Roopjote Atwal, Anthony Panasci, Emma Morris, and Allie Cho. Thank you to my Joburg research associate Lindile Cele and my mentees Edna Bosire and Andy Kim. And a special thank you to Emma Backe for giving an early version of this manuscript a critical and deep think.

Along the way, I was incredibly lucky to meet Zachary Gresham. He is funny, a critical reader, and an excellent editor who supported this book and for whom I could not be more thankful. Also, the co-editors of the Policy to Practice series with Vanderbilt University Press including Judith Justice, Peter J. Brown, and Svea Closser, are the most fun, thoughtful, committed, and knowledgeable group of scholars and friends.

Caring for my little ones amid the pandemic became lighter when Tyler Branford popped quite unexpectedly into our lives. Thank you for showering my little ones with love during the work day. The pandemic has been so hard for working families (especially moms), and this project would have been impossible without her finding us. We thank our lucky stars that she did.

A special thanks to Tom and Hannah Mullins and Christie Walser for sundowners and great feedback, and to Kate Giguere Morris for coming up with the title.

Finally, thank you to Adam, Fiona, and Zoë for filling my life with surprises. I feel lucky each and every day for having you in my life.

NOTES

PROLOGUE

1. I have called this lake "West Lake Okoboji" for my entire life, but the geological survey of the region calls it West Okoboji Lake. I use these names interchangeably throughout the book. Residents mostly refer to the lakes as West Lake Okoboji or East Lake Okoboji.
2. This work was described in my first book, *Syndemic Suffering: Social Distress, Depression, and Diabetes among Mexican Immigrant Women* (New York: Routledge, 2012).
3. This research was described in my second book, a meditation on a decade of collaborative work with colleagues around the world: *Rethinking Diabetes: Entanglements with Trauma, Poverty, and HIV* (Ithaca, NY: Cornell University Press, 2019).

CHAPTER 1

1. Alexandra L. Phelan, Rebecca Katz, and Lawrence O. Gostin, "The Novel Coronavirus Originating in Wuhan, China," *JAMA* 323, no. 8 (Jan. 30, 2020): 709–10, https://jamanetwork.com/journals/jama/fullarticle/2760500.
2. Steve Epstein, *Impure Science: AIDS, Activism, and the Politics of Knowledge* (Berkeley: University of California Press, 1998).
3. Michael Ryan, "Dr. Alfred Katz Says Fear, Not Aids, Is Causing a Red Cross Blood Loss," *People Magazine*, July 11, 1983, https://people.com/archive/dr-alfred-katz-says-fear-not-aids-is-causing-a-red-cross-blood-loss-vol-20-no-2.

4. Lisa A. Eaton and Seth C. Kalichman, "Social and Behavioral Health Responses to COVID-19: Lessons Learned from Four Decades of the HIV Pandemic," *Journal of Behavioral Medicine* 43, no. 3 (June 2020): 341–45. DOI: 10.1007/s10865-020-00157-y.

5. See Paul Farmer, *AIDS and Accusation: Haiti and the Geography of Blame* (Berkeley: University of California Press, 1992).

6. Albena Dzhurova, "Symbolic Politics and Government Response to a National Emergency: Narrating the COVID-19 Crisis," *Administrative Theory & Praxis* 42, no. 4 (2020): 571–87, DOI: 10.1080/10841806.2020.1816787.

7. Randy Schilts, *And the Band Played On: Politics, People, and the AIDS Epidemic* (New York: St. Martin's Griffin, 1987).

8. "Timeline of Trump's Coronavirus Responses," website of United States Congressman Lloyd Doggett, United States House of Representatives, January 20, 2021, https://doggett.house.gov/media-center/blog-posts/timeline-trump-s-coronavirus-responses.

9. Shilts, *And the Band Played On.*

10. Heidi Ledford, "Moderna COVID Vaccine Becomes Second to Get US Authorization: Two RNA Vaccines Will Be Useful as US Infections Surge, but the Speedy Authorizations Complicate Clinical Trials," *Nature*, Dec. 18, 2020, https://www.nature.com/articles/d41586-020-03593-7.

11. Randall Packard, *A History of Global Health: Interventions into the Lives of Other Peoples*, (Baltimore, MD: Johns Hopkins University Press, 2016); Owen Dyer, "Covid-19: Many Poor Countries Will See Almost No Vaccine Next Year, Aid Groups Warn," *BMJ*, no. 371 (Dec. 11, 2021): m2809, https://www.bmj.com/content/371/bmj.m4809; Dan Diamond, Tyler Pager, and Jeff Stein, "Biden Commits to Waiving Vaccine Patents, Driving Wedge with Pharmaceutical Companies," *Washington Post*, May 5, 2021, https://www.washingtonpost.com/health/2021/05/05/biden-wavies-vaccine-patents.

12. Paul Farmer, Arthur Kleinman, Jim Y. Kim, and Matthew Basilico, *Reimagining Global Health: An Introduction* (Berkeley:

University of California Press, 2013); Anne-Emanuelle Birn, Yogan Pillay, and Timothy Holtz, *Textbook of Global Health*, 4th ed. (Oxford, UK: Oxford University Press, 2017).

13. Barack Obama, "Remarks by the President at Cairo University, 6-04-09," The White House: President Barak Obama, archives, June 4, 2009, https://obamawhitehouse.archives.gov/the-press-office/remarks-president-cairo-university-6-04-09.

14. Julie Fischer and Rebecca Katz, "U.S. Priorities for Global Health Security," in *Global Health Policy in the Second Obama Term: A Report of the CSIS Global Health Policy Center*, ed., J. Stephen Morrison, 85–95 (Washington, DC: Global Health Policy Center, 2013).

15. Alexandra L. Phelan and Lawrence Gostin, "Law as a Fixture between the One Health Interfaces of Emerging Diseases," *Transactions of the Royal Society of Tropical Medicine and Hygiene* 111, no. 6 (2017): 241–43, doi: 10.1093/trstmh/trx044.

16. Lawrence Gostin and Rebecca Katz, "The International Health Regulations: The Governing Framework for Global Health Security," *Milbank Quarterly* 94, no. 2 (2016): 264–313.

17. Packard, *A History of Global Health.*

18. Jeremy Konyndyk, "Global Health Security in the Trump Era: Time to Worry?" *Commentary and Analysis* (blog), Center for Global Development, May 17, 2018, https://www.cgdev.org/blog/global-health-security-trump-era-time-worry.

19. Michael D. Lemonick and Alice Park, "The Truth about SARS," *Time*, May 5, 2003, http://content.time.com/time/subscriber/article/0,33009,1004763,00.html.

20. Elizabeth E. Cameron, Jennifer B. Nuzzo, and Jessica A. Bell, *Global Health Security Index: Building Collective Action and Accountability*, report (Washington, DC: Nuclear Threat Initiative, October 2019), https://www.ghsindex.org/wp-content/uploads/2020/04/2019-Global-Health-Security-Index.pdf.

21. "Timeline of Trump's Coronavirus Responses."

22. "Timeline: WHO's COVID-19 Response," World Health Organization, accessed Sept. 7, 2021, https://www.who.int/

emergencies/diseases/novel-coronavirus-2019/interactive-
timeline.

23. Peter Nicholas and Ed Yong, "Fauci: 'Bizarre' White House
Behavior Only Hurts the President," *The Atlantic*, July 15,
2020, https://www.theatlantic.com/politics/archive/2020/07/
trump-fauci-coronavirus-pandemic-oppo/614224.

24. Peter Nicholas and Kathy Gilsinan, "The End of the Imperial
Presidency," *The Atlantic*, May 2, 2020, https://www.theatlantic.
com/politics/archive/2020/05/trump-governors-coronavirus/
611023.

25. Eric Levitz, "Trump Condemns New York for Planning Ahead
on Coronavirus, *New York Magazine: Intelligencer*, March 30,
2020, https://nymag.com/intelligencer/2020/03/coronavi-
rus-trump-new-york-ventilators-cuomo.html.

26. Drew Altman, "Understanding the US Failure on Coronavirus—
An Essay by Drew Altman," *BMJ*, no. 370 (Sept. 14, 2020): m3417,
https://www.bmj.com/content/370/bmj.m3417.

27. Mega Molteni, "Iowa's Covid Wave and the Limits of Personal
Responsibility, *Wired*, November 20, 2020, https://www.wired.com/
story/iowas-covid-wave-and-the-limits-of-personal-responsibility.

28. Samuel Bazzi, Martin Fiszbein, and Mesay Gebresilasse, *Rugged
Individualism and Collective (In)Action During the COVID-19
Pandemic*, NBER Working Paper Series, vol. 5 (Cambridge, MA:
National Bureau of Economic Research, 2020), 2. https://www.
nber.org/papers/w27776.

29. Kristin L. Hoganson, *The Heartland: An American History* (New
York: Penguin Press, 2019), 136.

30. David P. Carter and Peter J. May, "Making Sense of the U.S.
COVID-19 Pandemic Response: A Policy Regime Perspective,"
Administrative Theory and Praxis 42, no. 2 (2020): 265–77.

CHAPTER 2

1. Lakes Regional Healthcare, "You've heard about it everywhere:
coronavirus," Facebook, March 9, 2020, https://www.facebook.
com/lakesregionalhealthcare/posts/10157130961737895.

2. Zach Borus, "COVID-19 Coronavirus Things to Know: 3/9/2020," lakeshealth (Lakes Regional Healthcare), YouYube video, March 9, 2020, https://youtu.be/ojy6hjfaODk.
3. Tedros Adhanom Ghebreyesus, "Acting on NCDs: Counting the Cost," *Lancet* 391, no. 10134 (May 19, 2018): 1973–73, https://doi.org/10.1016/S0140-6736(18)30675-5.
4. Congressman Adam Schiff, "Coronavirus Q&A: Rep. Schiff and Dr. Rebecca Katz," Facebook Live, March 12, 2020. https://www.facebook.com/RepAdamSchiff/videos/2300565436907522.
5. MPRNews Staff, Hannah Yang, "COVID-19 Cases Confirmed at SW Minn. Pork Processing Plant," *MPR News*, April 17, 2020, https://www.mprnews.org/story/2020/04/17/sw-minns-nobles-county-sees-jump-in-covid19-cases.
6. Dan Charles, "How One City Mayor Forced a Pork Giant to Close Its Virus-Stricken Plant," NPR, April 14, 2020, https://www.npr.org/2020/04/14/834470141/how-one-city-mayor-forced-a-pork-giant-to-close-its-virus-stricken-plant.
7. Renato Rosaldo, from a comment at Anthropology and "the Field": Boundaries, Areas, and Grounds in the Constitution of a Discipline conference held at Stanford University and UC Santa Cruz, February 18–19, 1994. See James Clifford, "Spatial Practices: Fieldwork, Travel, and the Disciplining of Anthropology," in *Anthropological Locations: Boundaries and Grounds of a Field Science*, edited by Akhil Gupta and James Ferguson (Berkeley: University of California Press, 1997), 219n2.
8. I reached out to study participants to request their participation over text, Facebook Messenger, email, and phone. Every study participant verbally consented to participate in an interview, and I recorded, transcribed, and analyzed our conversations. People I spoke to were mostly former classmates, friends, friends of friends, or people who reached out to me after they learned about my project. I also spoke with hundreds of people informally in person, online, and via text. This could have involved exchanges over Facebook Messenger or a masked conversation on the sidewalk at Arnolds Park where my kids were eat-

ing Nutty Bars—a tasty local treat of ice cream covered in frozen chocolate and nuts.

9. Erik H. Erikson, *Childhood and Society*, 2nd ed. (New York: Norton, 1993).

10. Gwen Westerman and Bruce White, *Mni Sota Makoce: The Land of the Dakota* (St Paul: Minnesota Historical Society Press, 2012), 13; quoted in Caroline Fraser, *Prairie Fires: The American Dreams of Laura Ingles Wilder* (New York: Metropolitan Books, 2017), 10.

11. For a widely accepted origin myth, see Hattie P. Elston, *White Men Follow After: A Collection of Stories about the Okoboji-Spirit Lake Region* (Spirit Lake, IA: Dickinson County Historical Society and Museum, 1988).

12. Abbie Gardner-Sharp, *History of the Spirit Lake Massacre and Captivity of Miss Abbie Gardner* (Des Moines, IA: Wallace-Homestead Book, 1885).

13. Fraser, *Prairie Fires*, 9–24.

14. Ibid.

15. Katie Prout, "A History of Violence: Walking the Blood-Soaked Shores of Spirit Lake: Rethinking an Early-American Captivity Narrative," *Literary Hub*, March 1, 2017, https://lithub.com/crime-or-conflict-walking-the-blood-soaked-shores-of-spirit-lake. This piece involves an interview with the longtime caretaker of the Abbie Gardner Cabin, Mike Koppert. Another relevant book is John Parsons, *Inkpaduta and the Sioux Indians* (Spirit Lake, IA: Okoboji Protective Association, 1998).

16. Gardner-Sharp, *History of the Spirit Lake Massacre*.

17. Fraser, *Prairie Fires*, 22.

18. Prout, "A History of Violence."

19. Some Dakota, Lakota, and Nakota are writing histories of settler colonialism. One great example is the Oak Lake Writers Society, Craig Howe, and Kim TallBear, eds., *This Stretch of River* (Sioux Falls, SD: Pine Hill Press, 2006).

20. Julie Zauzmer, "Following the Pittsburgh Attack, Rep. Steve King's Iowa Supporters Brush Aside Concern about His White

Nationalist Views," *Washington Post*, October 28, 2018, https://
www.washingtonpost.com/politics/in-the-wake-of-the-
pittsburgh-attack-rep-steve-kings-iowa-supporters-brush-aside-
concern-about-his-white-nationalist-views/2018/10/28/
a16b7044-dabf-11e8-b732-3c72cbf131f2_story.html.
21. "Dickinson County, IA," Data USA, accessed on November 9,
    2020, https://datausa.io/profile/geo/dickinson-county-ia.
22. "Emmet County, IA," Data USA, accessed on November 9, 2020,
    https://datausa.io/profile/geo/emmet-county-ia.
23. "Buena Vista County, IA," Data USA, accessed on November 9,
    2020, https://datausa.io/profile/geo/buena-vista-county-ia.
24. Hoganson, *The Heartland.*
25. Art Cullen, *Storm Lake: A Chronicle of Change, Resilience, and
    Hope from a Heartland Newspaper* (New York: Penguin Random
    House, 2018).
26. James Baldwin, "On Being 'White' . . . and Other Lies," in *Black
    on White: Black Writers on What It Means to Be White*, ed.,
    David R. Roediger, 177–80 (New York: Schocken Books, 1998).
27. Baldwin, "On Being 'White,'" 179–80.
28. Hoganson, *The Heartland.*
29. Hoganson, *The Heartland*, xxi
30. Sarah Smarsh, *Heartland: A Memoir of Working Hard and Being
    Broke in the Richest Country on Earth* (New York: Scribner,
    2019).
31. "Dickinson County, Iowa: 2020 General Election," Election
    Results, Scytl.us, last updated November 12, 2020, https://
    electionresults.iowa.gov/IA/Dickinson/106309.
32. Jonathan Haidt, *The Righteous Mind: Why Good People Are
    Divided by Politics and Religion* (New York: Vintage, 2012).
33. Nora Kenworthy, Adam Koon, and Emily Mendenhall, "On
    Symbols and Scripts: The Politics of the American COVID-19
    Response," *Global Public Health* 16, no. 8-9 (March 19, 2021):
    1424–38, DOI: 10.1080/17441692.2021.1902549.
34. Francis Fukuyama, *Identity: The Demand for Dignity and the
    Politics of Resentment* (New York: Farrar, Strauss, Giroux, 2018), 27.

35. Fukuyama, 40–41.
36. Fukuyama, 46.

CHAPTER 3

1. Amanda Moreland et al., "Timing of State and Territorial COVID-19 Stay-at-Home Orders and Changes in Population Movement— United States, March 1–May 31, 2020," *Morbidity and Mortality Weekly Report* 69, no. 35 (September 4, 2020): 1198–203, https://www.cdc.gov/mmwr/volumes/69/wr/mm6935a2.htm.
2. John Wills, "When Should Iowa Reopen the Economy?" *Dickinson County News*, April 28, 2020, https://www.dickinsoncountynews.com/story/2686550.html.
3. Unfortunately, the third brother passed away.
4. "University of Okoboji," Vacation Okoboji, accessed Aug. 18, 2021, https://vacationokoboji.com/about/university-of-okoboji.
5. "History," Berkley Fishing, accessed Aug. 18, 2021, https://www.berkley-fishing.com/pages/berkley-history.
6. Larry Ramey and Daniel Haley, *Tackling Giants: The Life Story of Berkley Bedell* (Loveland, CO: National Foundation of Alternative Medicine, 2005).
7. Ramey and Haley, *Tackling Giants*.
8. "Jarden Corporation Acquires Pure Fishing, Inc." Industry News Archive, Bass Resource, April 11, 2007, https://www.bassresource.com/bass_fishing_123/pure_fishing_sold_07.html.
9. City of Okoboji, Iowa, v Leo Parks, Jr. and Okoboji Barz, Inc. d/b/a Okoboji Boat Works, Fish House Lounge and Clucker's Broasted Chicken, 830 N.W.2nd 300 (Iowa Sup. 2013). https://www.iowacourts.gov/static/media/documents/120335_9DB20736237F2.pdf. ·
10. Russ Mitchell, "Iowa Supreme Court Issues 'Fish House Lounge' Ruling," *Dickinson County News*, April 26, 2013, https://siouxcityjournal.com/business/okoboji-businessman-files-lawsuit-against-city-council/article_86036b56-d53f-5ca4-a40c-ff7e167509c7.html; *City of Okoboji v Leo Parks, Jr.*

11. Seth Boyes, "DNR Votes Down Petition to Thin Millers Bay Boat Traffic," *Dickinson County News*, Nov. 17, 2020, https://www.dickinsoncountynews.com/story/2848481.html.

12. Michael J. Lanoo, *The Iowa Lakeside Laboratory: A Century of Discovering the Nature of Nature* (Iowa City: University of Iowa Press, 2012).

13. Seth Boyes, "We Don't Need No Nanny State," *Dickinson County News*, July 8, 2020, https://www.dickinsoncountynews.com/blogs/sethboyes/entry/75036.

14. "Iowa Great Lakes Walleye Weekend," Iowa Great Lakes Area Chamber of Commerce, accessed March 2, 2021, https://okobojichamber.com/walleye-weekend.

15. Personal communication, Iowa Great Lakes Chamber of Commerce, May 4, 2021.

16. Perhaps to promote tourism, the Iowa Lakes Chamber of Commerce set the prizes at $39,000 for 2021.

17. "Iowa Great Lakes Walleye Weekend," Iowa Great Lakes Area Chamber of Commerce, accessed March 2, 2021, https://okobojichamber.com/walleye-weekend.

18. "President Trump Meets with the Governor of Iowa," Trump White House Archived, YouTube video, May 6, 2020, https://www.youtube.com/watch?v=Ok1T1XMZaho.

19. Brianne Pfannenstiel and Nick Coltrain, "Gov. Kim Reynolds Says Iowa Will Loosen Restrictions on the Economy This Week," *Des Moines Register*, May 11, 2020, https://www.desmoinesregister.com/story/news/health/2020/05/11/iowa-gov-kim-reynolds-covid-19-coronavirus-data-matrix-maps-reopening/3073063001.

20. Brianne Pfannenstiel, and Nick Coltrain, "Iowa Gov. Kim Reynolds Taking Extra Precautions, State Epidemiologist Quarantining after Potential Coronavirus Exposure at White House," *Des Moines Register*, May 11, 2020, https://www.desmoinesregister.com/story/news/politics/2020/05/11/iowa-gov-reynolds-extra-precautions-white-house-visit-coronavirus-exposure-mike-pence/3106601001.

21. "Gov. Reynolds signs new proclamation continuing the State Public Health Emergency Declaration," Office of the Governor of

Iowa Kim Reynolds, May 20, 2020, https://governor.iowa.gov/
press-release/gov-reynolds-signs-new-proclamation-continuing-
the-state-public-health-emergency-3.

22. The Emporium was acquired by Parks Marina in 2016. "Parks
Marina Acquires Okoboji's Central Emporium," *Sioux Falls
Business Journal*, May 3, 2016, https://www.argusleader.com/
story/news/business-journal/2016/05/03/parks-marina-
acquires-okobojis-central-emporium/83820420.

23. Jeff Thee, "Okoboji Broadcast with Jeff Thee #78 – Debbie
Parks," Facebook, May 28, 2020, https://www.facebook.com/
watch/?v=268468074301807.

CHAPTER 4

1. Anne Lamott, *Bird by Bird: Some Instructions on Writing and
Life* (New York: Anchor Books, 1994).

2. Dargan Soutard, "Tyson Meat Plant in Storm Lake to Shut Down
Temporarily after State Confirms Coronavirus Outbreak," *Des
Moines Register*, May 28, 2020, https://www.desmoinesregister.
com/story/news/politics/2020/05/28/coronavirus-outbreak-
confirmed-tyson-foods-storm-lake-pork-processing-plant-
kim-reynolds/5274618002.

3. Lanoo, *The Iowa Lakeside Laboratory*.

4. Evan Coughlin, "Three SC Metropolitan Areas Currently among
Top 30 Hot Spots in America for COVID-19," WIS News, June 16,
2020, https://www.wistv.com/2020/06/16/three-sc-metropolitan-
areas-currently-among-top-hot-spots-america-covid-; Emily
Mendenhall, "How an Iowa Summer Resort Region Became
a Covid-19 Hot Spot," Vox, August 8, 2020, https://www.vox.
com/2020/8/8/21357625/covid-19-iowa-lakes-okoboji-kim-
reynolds-masks.

CHAPTER 5

1. Seth Boyes, "Ernst Checks on Local Health Needs during Pandemic," *Dickinson County News*, July 14, 2020, https://www.
dickinsoncountynews.com/story/2822665.html.

2. Lenore Manderson and Susan Levine, "COVID-19, Risk, Fear, and Fall-Out," *Medical Anthropology* 39 no. 5 (2020): 369.

3. Although Clay County calls its county fair *the largest county fair* in the nation, many other counties in other states think theirs is also the biggest in the nation.

4. Millissa Reynolds, Okoboji Barz, Inc., is a member of the board. "Iowa Restaurant Association Board of Directors," Iowa Restaurant Association, accessed Sept. 10, 2021, https://restaurantiowa.com/board-of-directors.

5. Gavin Aronsen, "The Businesspeople Who Have Helped Enable Steve King's Rise: Part 2," *Iowa Informer*, February 23, 2019, http://iowainformer.com/politics/2019/02/steve-king-sukup-okoboji-caseys-kum-go-hepar.

6. Jonathan Grieder et al., "COVID-19 Response Should Protect Working Communities. Why Is the Governor Putting Corporate Profits First?," *Des Moines Register*, July 6, 2020, https://www.desmoinesregister.com/story/opinion/columnists/iowa-view/2020/07/06/local-iowa-officials-reynolds-has-wrong-priorities-covid-19-response/5360779002.

7. This was confirmed by personal communication with a patron; the Barefoot Cam can be accessed from the "Webcams" page of the Parks Marina website: https://www.parksmarina.com/webcams.

8. "Sirens 09-30-20: Local Business Cited for Inadequate COVID-19 Mitigation," *Dickinson County News*, September 29, 2020, https://www.dickinsoncountynews.com/story/2838120.html.

9. This was confirmed by a personal communication with someone invited to the event.

10. Carter and May, "Making Sense of the U.S. COVID-19 Pandemic Response," 273.

11. Charles L. Briggs and Clara Matini-Briggs, *Stories in the Time of Cholera: Racial Profiling during a Medical Nightmare* (Berkeley: University of California Press, 2003), 47.

12. CNN Wire, "U.S. Coronavirus Cases Top 6 Million as Birx Urges Americans 'Do the Right Thing' to Slow Spread," KTLA 5, Nexstar Media, August 31, 2020, https://ktla.com/news/

coronavirus/u-s-coronavirus-cases-near-6-million-as-dr-birx-urges-americans-to-do-the-right-thing-and-slow-the-spread.

13. See John Wills, "It's Time to Return Lost Rights," *Dickinson County News*, May 19, 2020, https://www.dickinsoncountynews.com/story/2810675.html.

14. Elaine Godfrey, "Iowa Is What Happens When Government Does Nothing," *The Atlantic*, Dec. 3, 2020, https://www.theatlantic.com/politics/archive/2020/12/how-iowa-mishandled-coronavirus-pandemic/617252.

CHAPTER 6

1. Annemarie Mol, *The Logic of Care: Health and the Problem of Patient Choice* (New York: Routledge, 2008).

2. Fukuyama, *Identity*, 10–11.

3. Jonathan Metzl, *Dying of Whiteness: How the Politics of Racial Resentment Is Killing America's Heartland* (New York: Basic Books, 2019), 52.

4. Eden Litt and Eszter Hargittai, "The Imagined Audience on Social Network Sites," *Social Media + Society* 2, no. 1 (January–March 2016): 1–12; also see Zizi Papacharissi, *Affective Publics: Sentiment, Technology, and Politics* (Oxford, UK: Oxford University Press, 2014).

5. Naseem Ahmed et al., "The COVID-19 Infodemic: A Quantitative Analysis through Facebook," *Cureus* 12, no. 11 (2020), https://doi.org/10.7759/cureus.11346.

6. "The COVD-19 Infodemic," *Lancet Infectious Diseases* 20, no. 8 (Aug. 2020): 875.

7. Seth Boyes, "LRH Confirms First COVID-19 Death in Dickson County," *Dickinson County News*, June 15, 2020, https://www.dickinsoncountynews.com/story/2816631.html.

8. Seth Boyes, "Maxwell's Beach Café Takes Voluntary Two-Week Break as COVID-19 Cases Rise," *Dickinson County News*, June 12, 2020, https://www.dickinsoncountynews.com/story/2816361.html.

9. Maxwell's Beach Café. "UPDATE: On Thursday, Dickinson County Board of Health and Lakes Regional Healthcare

reported" Facebook, June 11, 2020, https://www.facebook.com/ maxwellsbeachcafe/posts/3533509353344710.

10. Kenworthy, Koon, and Mendenhall, "On Symbols and Scripts."

11. Kenworthy, Koon, and Mendenhall, "On Symbols and Scripts."

12. "Vaccine Safety: Autism and Vaccines." Centers for Disease Control and Prevention, last reviewed August 25, 2020, https:// www.cdc.gov/vaccinesafety/concerns/autism.html.

13. See Wills, "It's Time to Return Lost Rights."

14. Matthew Sparke and Dimitar Anguelov, "Contextualising Coronavirus Geographically," *Transactions of the Institute of British Geographers* 45, no. 3 (Sept. 2020): 498–508.

15. "The Story," Okoboji Store, accessed Aug. 20, 2021, https:// theokobojistore.com/story.

CHAPTER 7

1. Claude Lévi-Strauss, *The Savage Mind* (Chicago: University of Chicago Press, 1966), first published as *La Pensée sauvage* (Paris: Librairie Plon, 1962).

2. Jason Kirschbaum, "Living it up at our place," Facebook, June 7, 2020, https://www.facebook.com/profile. php?id=100024182986609.

3. Mol, *The Logic of Care*, 7.

4. After I returned to the Washington, DC, area in August, however, I began wearing a mask at all times. This was in part because masking recommendations changed with the fall virus surge and people were encouraged to wear masks inside and outside. But it was also because, when I was at the Lakes, nobody wore masks outside. When I arrived back in DC, everyone did; I was shamed outright when running without a mask in DC in early September. I never made that mistake again.

5. Adam Grant, "There's a Name for the Blah You're Feeling: It's Called Languishing," *New York Times*, April 19, 2021, https:// www.nytimes.com/2021/04/19/well/mind/covid-mental-health-languishing.html.

6. Matthew Cohen, "The Rise in Testing Is Not Driving the Rise in U.S. Virus Cases," *New York Times*, July 22, 2020, https://www. nytimes.com/interactive/2020/07/22/us/covid-testing-rising-cases.html.

CHAPTER 8

1. Don Gonyea, "'God Bless the U.S.A.,' A Country Anthem with Enduring Political Power," *NPR Morning Edition*, Sept. 11, 2018, https://www.npr.org/2018/09/11/645270955/god-bless-the-u-s-a-a-country-anthem-with-enduring-political-power.
2. Gonyea, "'God Bless the U.S.A.'"
3. Arvin Temkar, "My Fellow Liberals Hate Lee Greenwood's 'God Bless the USA.'; I Love It," *Washington Post*, June 30, 2017, https://www.washingtonpost.com/outlook/my-fellow-liberals-hate-lee-greenwoods-god-bless-the-usa-i-love-it/2017/06/30/e09ce46a-5a9f-11e7-9fc6-c7ef4bc58d13_story.html.
4. Lee Greenwood, "God Bless the U.S.A." *You've Got a Good Love Comin'*, MCA Records, 1984.
5. Greenwood, "God Bless the U.S.A."
6. "Douglas Alexander, 67, Arnolds Park," obituary, N'West Iowa, https://www.nwestiowa.com/obituaries/douglas-alexander-67-arnolds-park/article_1b2190ce-bfd1-11ea-883e-a3009e221d74. html.
7. The arrivalist methodology counts "travelers that have traveled at least 50 miles from home, spent a minimum of two hours in Iowa, spent up to 14 days in Iowa to be counted as a completed round trip, includes adults 18+, U.S. visitors only, excludes commuters, devices include regular GPS pings and smartphone users only"; "Arrivalist Dashboard," Travel Iowa, accessed Sept. 9, 2021, https://www. traveliowa.com/industry-partners/research/arrivalist-dashboard.
8. Katie Peikes, "Okoboji's Summer Tourism Season Drew Fewer Visitors Because of the Pandemic," Iowa Public Radio News, September 8, 2020, https://www.iowapublicradio.org/ipr-news/2020-09-08/okobojis-summer-tourism-season-drew-fewer-visitors-because-of-pandemic.

9. Camp Foster YMCA, "A big part of our camp programming is teaching kids skills," Facebook, June 24, 2020, https://www.facebook.com/campfosterYMCA/posts/10159133640217366.
10. Nick Hytek, "COVID-19 Trends Rise across State, but not in Northwest Iowa," *Sioux City Journal*, July 25, 2020, https://siouxcityjournal.com/news/local/covid-19-trends-rise-across-state-but-not-in-northwest-iowa/article_f15b5058-87db-5b8b-8531-ec14c8d98fcc.html.

1. Brynne Keith-Jennings, "Food Need Very High Compared to Pre-Pandemic Levels, Making Relief Imperative," *Off the Charts* (blog), Center on Budget and Policy Priorities, Sept. 10, 2020, https://www.cbpp.org/blog/food-need-very-high-compared-to-pre-pandemic-levels-making-relief-imperative.
2. "Tracking the COVID-19 Recession's Effects on Food, Housing, and Employment Hardships," Center on Budget and Policy Priorities, Feb. 11, 2021, https://www.cbpp.org/research/poverty-and-inequality/tracking-the-covid-19-recessions-effects-on-food-housing-and.
3. Lawrence Michel et al., *The State of Working America*, 12th ed. (Ithaca, NY: Economic Policy Institute book published by Cornell University Press, 2012), http://www.stateofworkingamerica.org/subjects/income/index.html.
4. David L. Blustein and Paige A. Guarina, "Work and Unemployment in the Time of COVID-19: The Existential Experience of Loss and Fear," *Journal of Humanistic Psychology* 60, no. 5 (2020): 702–9.
5. Julie Kashen, Sarah Jane Glynn, and Amanda Novello, "How COVID-19 Sent Women's Workforce Progress Backward," Center for American Progress, October 30, 2020, https://www.americanprogress.org/issues/women/reports/2020/10/30/492582/covid-19-sent-womens-workforce-progress-backward.
6. Thurka Sangaramoorthy and Adia Benton, "Imagining Rural Immunity," *Anthropology News*, June 19, 2020, https://www.

anthropology-news.org/index.php/2020/06/19/imagining-
rural-immunity; Bradley L. Hardy and Trevon D. Logan,
Racial Economic Inequality amid the COVID-19 Crisis, The
Hamilton Project, Essay 2020-17 (Washington, DC: Brookings,
August 2020), https://www.brookings.edu/wp-content/
uploads/2020/08/EA_HardyLogan_LO_8.12.pdf.

7. Kenworthy, Koon, and Mendenhall, "On Symbols and Scripts."

8. Metzl, *Dying of Whiteness*, 5.

9. Metzl, *Dying of Whiteness*, 8.

10. Christian Paz, "All the President's Lies about the Coronavirus:
An Unfinished Compendium of Trump's Overwhelming
Dishonesty during a National Emergency," *The Atlantic*, Nov. 2,
2020, https://www.theatlantic.com/politics/archive/2020/11/
trumps-lies-about-coronavirus/608647.

11. Walmart put this national mask-wearing policy in place on July
20, 2020. "A Simple Step to Help Keep You Safe: Walmart and
Sam's Club Require Shoppers to Wear Face Coverings," Walmart
Corporate, July 15, 2020, https://corporate.walmart.com/newsroom/
2020/07/15/a-simple-step-to-help-keep-you-safe-walmart-and-
sams-club-require-shoppers-to-wear-face-coverings.

12. Adam Reich and Peter Bearman, *Working for Respect:
Community and Conflict at Walmart* (Ithaca, NY: Columbia
University Press, 2018).

13. Cullen, *Storm Lake*.

14. Olga Khazan, "How a Bizarre Claim about Masks Has Lived
on for Months," *The Atlantic*, Oct. 9, 2020, https://www.the-
atlantic.com/politics/archive/2020/10/can-masks-make-you-
sicker/616641.

15. Jennifer Senior, "I Spoke with Anthony Fauci. He Says His Inbox
Isn't Pretty," *New York Times*, July 21, 2020, https://www.nytimes.
com/2020/07/21/opinion/anthony-fauci-coronavirus.html.

16. Metzl, *Dying of Whiteness*, 10; italics in original.

17. Kimberly Amadeo, "Why Trickle-Down Economics Works
in Theory but Not in Fact: The Shortcomings of Supply-Side
Economics," *The Balance*, updated Jan. 21, 2021, https://www.

thebalance.com/trickle-down-economics-theory-effect-does-it-
work-3305572.

18. Runya Qiaoan, "The Myth of Masks: A Tale of Risk Selection in
the COVID-19 Pandemic," "Forum on COVID-19 Pandemic," special issue of *Social Anthropology* 28, no. 2 (May 2020): 336–37,
https://onlinelibrary.wiley.com/doi/10.1111/1469-8676.12852.

CHAPTER 10

1. Kristin Brig, "Anti-Vax to Anti-Mask: Processing Anti-Science
Claims during a Pandemic," *Biomedical Odyssey: Life at the Johns
Hopkins School of Medicine* (blog), Sept. 3, 2020, https://
biomedicalodyssey.blogs.hopkinsmedicine.org/2020/09/anti-vax-
to-anti-mask-processing-anti-science-claims-during-a-pandemic.

2. Jonathan M. Berman, *Anti-Vaxxers: How to Challenge a
Misinformed Movement* (Boston, MA: MIT Press, 2020); Heidi
Larson, *Stuck: How Vaccine Rumors Start—and Why They Don't
Go Away* (Oxford, UK: Oxford University Press, 2020).

3. Laura Eggertson, "Lancet Retracts 12-Year-Old Article Linking
Autism to MMR Vaccines," *Canadian Medical Association
Journal* 182, no. 4 (2010): E199–E200; A. Wakefield et al.,
"RETRACTED: Ileal-Lymphoid-Nodular Hyperplasia, Non-
Specific Colitis, and Pervasive Developmental Disorder in
Children." *Lancet* 351, no. 9103 (1998): 637–41.

4. Larson, *Stuck.*

5. Larson, 124

6. Jennifer Reich, "Neoliberal Mothering and Vaccine Refusal:
Imagined Gated Communities and the Privilege of Choice,"
Gender & Society 28, no. 5 (2014): 679–704.

7. Jennifer Reich, "'We Are Fierce, Independent Thinkers and
Intelligent': Social Capital and Stigma Management among
Mothers Who Refuse Vaccines." *Social Science and Medicine* 257
(July 2020): 112015.

8. Khazan, "How a Bizarre Claim."

9. See Johnny Edwards, "Some Chiropractors Stoke Fear of Covid
Vaccine," *Seattle Times*, May 24, 2021, https://www.seattletimes.

com/seattle-news/health/some-chiropractors-stoking-fear-of-covid-vaccines. Some of this can be understood by the financial interest in promoting natural cure-alls. Geoff Brumfiel, "For Some Anti-Vaccine Advocates, Misinformation Is Part of a Business," NPR, May 21, 2021, https://www.npr.org/sections/health-shots/2021/05/12/993615185/for-some-anti-vaccine-advocates-misinformation-is-part-of-a-business.

10. Elisa J. Sobo, "Theorizing (Vaccine) Refusal: Through the Looking Glass," *Cultural Anthropology* 31, no. 3 (2016): 342–50.

11. "Vaccine Safety: Autism and Vaccines," Center for Disease Control and Prevention, last reviewed Aug. 25, 2020, https://www.cdc.gov/vaccinesafety/concerns/autism.html; Joel Rose, "Even If It's 'Bonkers,' Poll Finds Many Believe QAnon and Other Conspiracy Theories," NPR, Dec. 30, 2020, https://www.npr.org/2020/12/30/951095644/even-if-its-bonkers-poll-finds-many-believe-qanon-and-other-conspiracy-theories.

12. EJ Sobo, "Playing with Conspiracy Theories," *Anthropology News*, July 31, 2019, https://doi.org/10.1111/AN.1236.

13. Reich, "Neoliberal Mothering," 695.

14. Philip Smith, Susan Chu, and Lawrence Barker, "Children Who Have Received No Vaccines: Who Are They and Where Do They Live?," *Pediatrics* 114, no. 1 (July 2004): 187–95, DOI: https://doi.org/10.1542/peds.114.1.187.

15. Paul A. Djupe and Ryan P. Burge, "Trump the Anointed?," *Religion in Public: Exploring the Mix of Sacred and Secular* (blog), May 11, 2020, https://religioninpublic.blog/2020/05/11/trump-the-anointed.

16. On the website of the church this community attends—Downtown Church—they honor a perceived direct bond with God, a deepening of their values and beliefs, and co-dependence among their community (as their website describes, sharing "time, spiritual gifts, talents and money"). See more here: "Core Values of Downtown Church," accessed Aug. 23, 2021, http://media.wix.com/ugd/53dbfa_b2a3fa60bf40d650a77af9adb598a14b.pdf.

17. "Welcome to Downtown Church," Downtown Church, accessed February 10, 2021, https://www.downtownchurch.info.

18. Laura Ungar, "More Women Than Men Are Getting COVID Vaccines," *Scientific American*, April 12, 2021, https://www.scientificamerican.com/article/more-women-than-men-are-getting-covid-vaccines.

19. Cary Funk and Alec Tyson, "Growing Share of Americans Say They Plan to Get a COVID-19 Vaccine—or Already Have," Pew Research Center, March 5, 2021, https://www.pewresearch.org/science/2021/03/05/growing-share-of-americans-say-they-plan-to-get-a-covid-19-vaccine-or-already-have.

20. Yamiche Alcindor, "Why 41 Percent of Republicans Don't Plan to Get the COVID Vaccine," *PBS NewsHour*, March 19, 2021, https://www.pbs.org/newshour/show/why-41-percent-of-republicans-dont-plan-to-get-the-covid-vaccine.

21. Elizabeth Dias and Ruth Graham, "White Evangelical Resistance Is Obstacle in Vaccine Effort," *New York Times*, April 12, 2021, https://www.nytimes.com/2021/04/05/us/covid-vaccine-evangelicals.html.

22. Kevin Roose, "What Is QAnon, the Viral Pro-Trump Conspiracy Theory?" *New York Times*, Feb. 4, 2021, https://www.nytimes.com/article/what-is-qanon.html; "China Coronavirus: Misinformation Spreads Online about Origin and Scale," *BBC Trending* (blog), BBC News, Jan. 30, 2020, https:/www.bbc.com/news/blogs-trending-51271037.

23. Christen A. Smith, "Facing the Dragon: Black Mothering, Sequelae, and Gendered Necropolitics in the Americas." *Transforming Anthropology* 24, no. 1 (2016): 31–48; Lauren D. Nephew, "Systemic Racism and Overcoming My COVID-19 Vaccine Hesitancy," *EClinicalMedicine* 32 (Feb. 1, 2021): 100713, https://doi.org/10.1016/j.eclinm.2020.100713.

24. Elisa J. Sobo, "Social Cultivation of Vaccine Refusal and Delay among Waldorf (Steiner) School Parents," *Medical Anthropology Quarterly* 29, no. 3 (2015): 381–99.

25. Reuters Staff, "Fact Check: COVID-19 Vaccines Won't Alter Recipient DNA; Frontline Workers Have Suffered Directly from the Virus." Reuters, December 18, 2020, https://www.reuters.com/article/uk-factcheck-viral-post/fact-check-covid-19-vaccines-wont-alter-recipient-dna-frontline-workers-have-suffered-directly-from-the-virus-idUSKBN28S2V1; Flora Carmichael and Jack Goodman, "Vaccine Rumours Debunked: Microchips, 'Altered DNA' and More," Reality Check, BBC News, December 2, 2020, https://www.bbc.com/news/54893437.
26. For more on medical myths and pseudoscience, see Seema Yasmin, *Viral BS: Medical Myths and Why We Fall for Them* (Baltimore, MD: Johns Hopkins University Press, 2021).

CHAPTER 11

1. Molly Duffy, "Gov. Kim Reynolds Orders Iowa Schools to 'Take All Efforts' to Get Kids Back in Classrooms," *Gazette* (Iowa), July 17, 2020, https://www.thegazette.com/subject/news/education/gov-kim-reynolds-to-direct-all-iowa-schools-to-reopen-in-person-when-school-year-begins-next-month-20200717.
2. Duffy, "Gov. Kim Reynolds Orders Iowa schools."
3. Sharon Begley, "Trump Said More COVID-19 Testing 'Creates More Cases.' We Did the Math," STAT, July 20, 2020, https://www.statnews.com/2020/07/20/trump-said-more-covid19-testing-creates-more-cases-we-did-the-math.
4. Contact tracing, as defined by the CDC, is a case investigation that is central to the process of identifying who the patients with suspected or confirmed infection were in close contact with during the time frame in which they may have been infectious. This is usually done by public health staff using methods such as calling exposed individuals and asking about their exposure. "Case Investigation and Contact Tracing: Part of a Multipronged Approach to Fight the COVID-19 Pandemic," CDC, updated Dec. 3, 2020, https://www.cdc.gov/coronavirus/2019-ncov/php/principles-contact-tracing.html.

5. Brian Downing, "I have avoided joining in this discussion," Facebook, July 23, 2020, https://www.facebook.com/brian. downing.56/posts/10223875999596768.

6. This author of this post eventually deleted it; however, several people snapped screenshots of the post and shared them with me.

7. "School Responses to the Coronavirus (COVID-19) Pandemic during the 2020–2021 Academic Year," Ballotpedia, accessed May 11, 2021, https://ballotpedia.org/School_responses_to_the_ coronavirus_(COVID-19)_pandemic_during_the_2020-2021_ academic_year.

CHAPTER 12

1. Kimberly Frodl, "Debunked Myths about Face Masks," *Hometown Health* (blog), Mayo Clinic, July 10, 2020, https://www. mayoclinichealthsystem.org/hometown-health/speaking-of-health/debunked-myths-about-face-masks.

2. See Explore Okoboji for more discussion: "Spirit Lake School Bd Discusses Preparations for Start of School & COVID-19 Protocols," Explore Okoboji, August 3, 2020, https://www. exploreokoboji.com/news/news-stories/spirit-lake-school-bd-discusses-preparations-for-start-of-school-covid-19-protocols.

3. "'The Skunk at the Picnic': Dr. Anthony Fauci on Working for Trump," The Daily, *New York Times*, Jan. 26, 2021, https://www. nytimes.com/2021/01/26/podcasts/the-daily/anthony-fauci-donald-trump-coronavirus-pandemic.html.

CHAPTER 13

1. Mendenhall, "How an Iowa Summer Resort."

2. Richard Ashby, "My boyfriend and I just got harassed for wearing masks," Facebook, July 4, 2020.

3. Scott Van Aartsen, "Trump Parade Draws 'Hundreds' of Boats on West Okoboji," KIWA Radio, Aug. 8, 2020, https://kiwaradio. com/local-news/trump-parade-draws-hundreds-of-boats-on-west-okoboji.

CHAPTER 14

1. Seth Boyes, "Spirit Lake School Board Mandates Masks in Halls, Buses, not Classes," *Dickinson County News*, Aug. 11, 2020, https://www.dickinsoncountynews.com/story/2827994.html.
2. Ryan Foley, "'Horrifying' Data Glitch Skews Key Iowa Coronavirus Metrics," *Gazette* (Iowa), Aug. 17, 2020, https://www.thegazette.com/subject/news/government/iowa-covid-data-glitch-metrics-schools-percent-positive-20200817.
3. Ryan Foley, "Iowa Governor's Push to Reopen Schools Descends into Chaos," *AP News*, Iowa City, Aug. 19, 2020, https://apnews.com/article/319e899fe751d462fe3576c4010fb642.
4. Maeve Reston, "Donald Trump's Mind-Bending Logic on School Reopenings," CNN Politics, July 25, 2020, https://www.cnn.com/2020/07/25/politics/donald-trump-schools-reopening-coronavirus/index.html.
5. Foley, "'Horrifying' Data Glitch."
6. Tony Leys, "Gov. Kim Reynolds Says Iowans Can Trust State's Coronavirus Data, Despite History of Glitches," *Des Moines Register*, September 2, 2020, https://www.desmoinesregister.com/story/news/health/2020/09/02/governor-kim-reynolds-iowa-covid-19-data-trustworthy-despite-glitches/5695310002.
7. Tony Leys and Stephen Gruber-Miller, "Kim Reynolds Defends Iowa's COVID Data Credibility, Claims Transparency after 'Glitch' Skewed Official Numbers," *Des Moines Register*, Aug. 20, 2020, https://www.desmoinesregister.com/story/news/health/2020/08/20/iowa-health-leaders-fix-backdating-glitch-coronavirus-data-reports/5612558002.
8. Caroline Cummings, "After Glitch Fix, Experts Still Have Questions about State Coronavirus Data," *Iowa News Now*, Aug. 26, 2020, https://cbs2iowa.com/news/local/after-glitch-fix-experts-still-have-questions-about-state-coronavirus-data.

CHAPTER 15

1. Doug Woulter, "Sibley-Ocheyedan Football Team Battles Coronavirus, Hopes To Forge Winning Tradition," *Globe* (Worthington,

MN), Sept. 30, 2020, https://www.dglobe.com/sports/ 6681654-Sibley-Ocheyedan-football-team-battles-coronavirus-hopes-to-forge-winning-tradition.

2. Seth Boyes, "County to Vote on Mask Proclamation Next Week," *Dickinson County News*, Nov. 24, 2020, https://www. dickinsoncountynews.com/story/2849959.html.
3. Boyes, "County to Vote."
4. Boyes, "County to Vote."
5. Lindh Ta, "Reynolds Shifts Tone, Requires Masks Indoor as Hospitalizations Skyrocket," *Iowa Capital Dispatch*, Nov. 16, 2020, https://iowacapitaldispatch.com/2020/11/16/ reynolds-shifts-tone-requires-masks-indoor-as-hospitalizations-skyrocket.
6. Seth Boyes, "'It's Not a Mandate'—County Encourages Public Masking amid Pandemic," *Dickinson County News*, Dec. 1, 2020, https://www.dickinsoncountynews.com/story/2851073.html.
7. "Some Winter Games Traditions Continue, Others Paused until 2022," *Dickinson County News*, Jan. 12, 2020, https://www. dickinsoncountynews.com/story/2859316.html.
8. State of Iowa, Executive Department, "Proclamation of Disaster Emergency," February 5, 2021, https://governor.iowa. gov/sites/default/files/documents/Public%20Health%20 Proclamation%20-%202021.02.05.pdf.
9. "Positive Case Analysis," COVID-19 in Iowa, accessed May 18, 2021, https://coronavirus.iowa.gov/pages/case-counts; "COVID-19 Status Report," Johns Hopkins University Coronavirus Tracker, Iowa, Dickinson County, accessed June 2, 2021, https://bao. arcgis.com/covid-19/jhu/county/19059.html.
10. "See How Vaccinations Are Going in Your County and State," *New York Times*, accessed May 18, 2021, https.//www.nytimes. com/interactive/2020/us/covid-19-vaccine-doses.html.
11. Seth Boyes, "Local Schools Amend COVID-19 Policies," *Dickinson County News*, May 4, 2021, https://www. dickinsoncountynews.com/story/2881633.html.
12. "Okoboji's Downing Is Iowa Secondary Principal of the Year," School Administrators of Iowa, March 26, 2021, http://www.

sai-iowa.org/news.cfm/Article/News/Okobojis-Downing-is-
Iowa-Secondary-Principal-of-the-Year.

EPILOGUE

1. Agnes Binagwaho, "We Need Compassionate Leadership Management Based on Evidence to Defeat COVID-19," *International Journal of Health Policy and Management* 9, no. 10 (2020): 413–14; Eli M. Cahan, "Rwanda's Secret Weapon against COVID-19: Trust," *BMJ*, no. 371 (Dec. 11, 2020), https://www.bmj.com/content/371/bmj.m4720.
2. Nanjala Nyabola, "How to Talk about COVID-19 in Africa," *Boston Review*, Oct. 15, 2020, https://bostonreview.net/global-justice/nanjala-nyabola-how-talk-about-covid-19-africa.
3. Matt Kirstoffersen, "Planning for a Pandemic: A Biden COVID-19 Advisor Shares Perspective," Yale School of Public Health, March 3, 2021, https://publichealth.yale.edu/news-article/30725.
4. Rachel Blacher, "Commentary: An Ex-Pat Atlantan and Former CDC Staffer on What We Could Learn from Nearly Coronavirus-Free New Zealand," *Atlanta Magazine*, June 24, 2020, https://www.atlantamagazine.com/news-culture-articles/commentary-an-ex-pat-atlantan-and-former-cdc-staffer-on-what-we-could-learn-from-coronavirus-free-new-zealand.
5. Suze Wilson, "Three Reasons Why Jacinda Ardern's Coronavirus Response Has Been a Masterclass in Crisis Leadership," *The Conversation*, April 5, 2020, http://theconversation.com/three-reasonswhy-jacinda-arderns-coronavirus-response-has-been-a-masterclass-in-crisis-leadership-135541.

BIBLIOGRAPHY

Ahmed, Naseem, Tooba Shahbaz, Asma Shamim, Kiran Shafiq Khan,
  S. M. Hussain, and Asad Usman. "The COVID-19 Infodemic: A
  Quantitative Analysis through Facebook." *Cureus* 12, no. 11 (2020):
  e11346. https://doi.org/10.7759/cureus.11346.
Altman, Drew. "Understanding the US Failure on Coronavirus—An
  Essay by Drew Altman." *BMJ*, no. 370 (Sept. 14, 2020): m3417.
  https://www.bmj.com/content/370/bmj.m3417.
Amadeo, Kimberly. "Why Trickle-Down Economics Works in
  Theory but Not in Fact: The Shortcomings of Supply-Side
  Economics." *The Balance*, updated Jan. 21, 2021. https://www.
  thebalance.com/trickle-down-economics-theory-effect-does-it-
  work-3305572.
Baldwin, James. "On Being 'White' . . . and Other Lies." In *Black on
  White: Black Writers on What It Means To Be White*, edited by
  David R. Roediger, 177–80. New York: Schocken Books, 1998.
Bazzi, Samuel, Martin Fiszbein, and Mesay Gebresilasse. *Rugged
  Individualism and Collective (In)Action During the COVID-19
  Pandemic*. NBER Working Paper Series, vol. 5. Cambridge, MA:
  National Bureau of Economic Research, 2020. https://www.nber.
  org/papers/w27776.
Berman, Jonathan M. *Anti-Vaxxers: How to Challenge a Misin-
  formed Movement*. Boston, MA: MIT Press, 2020.
Binagwaho, Agnes. "We Need Compassionate Leadership Manage-
  ment Based on Evidence to Defeat COVID-19." *International*

Journal of Health Policy and Management 9, no. 10 (2020): 413–14.

Birn, Anne-Emanuelle, Yogan Pillay, and Timothy H. Holtz. *Textbook of Global Health*, 4th ed. Oxford, UK: Oxford University Press, 2017.

Blacher, Rachel. "Commentary: An Ex-Pat Atlantan and Former CDC Staffer on What We Could Learn from Nearly Coronavirus-Free New Zealand." *Atlanta Magazine*, June 24, 2020. https://www.atlantamagazine.com/news-culture-articles/commentary-an-ex-pat-atlantan-and-former-cdc-staffer-on-what-we-could-learn-from-coronavirus-free-new-zealand.

Blustein, David L., and Paige A. Guarina. "Work and Unemployment in the Time of COVID-19: The Existential Experience of Loss and Fear." *Journal of Humanistic Psychology* 60, no. 5 (2020): 702–9.

Boyes, Seth. "Maxwell's Beach Café Takes Voluntary Two-Week Break as COVID-19 Cases Rise." *Dickinson County News*, June 12, 2020. https://www.dickinsoncountynews.com/story/2816361.html.

Boyes, Seth. "LRH Confirms First COVID-19 Death in Dickson County." *Dickinson County News*, June 15, 2020. https://www.dickinsoncountynews.com/story/2816631.html.

Boyes, Seth. "We Don't Need No Nanny State." *Dickinson County News*, July 8, 2020. https://www.dickinsoncountynews.com/blogs/sethboyes/entry/75036.

Boyes, Seth. "Ernst Checks on Local Health Needs during Pandemic." *Dickinson County News*, July 14, 2020. https://www.dickinsoncountynews.com/story/2822665.html.

Boyes, Seth. "Spirit Lake School Board Mandates Masks in Halls, Buses, Not Classes." *Dickinson County News*, Aug. 11, 2020. https://www.dickinsoncountynews.com/story/2827994.html.

Boyes, Seth. "DNR Votes Down Petition to Thin Millers Bay Boat Traffic." *Dickinson County News*, Nov. 17, 2020. https://www.dickinsoncountynews.com/story/2848481.html.

Boyes, Seth. "County to Vote on Mask Proclamation Next Week." *Dickinson County News*, Nov. 24, 2020. https://www.dickinsoncountynews.com/story/2849959.html.

Boyes, Seth. "'It's Not a Mandate'—County Encourages Public Masking amid Pandemic." *Dickinson County News*, Dec. 1, 2020. https://www.dickinsoncountynews.com/story/2851073.html.

Boyes, Seth. "Local Schools Amend COVID-19 Policies." *Dickinson County News*, May 4, 2021. https://www.dickinsoncountynews.com/story/2881633.html.

Briggs, Charles L., and Clara Matini-Briggs. *Stories in the Time of Cholera: Racial Profiling during a Medical Nightmare*. Berkeley: University of California Press, 2003.

Cahan, Eli M. "Rwanda's Secret Weapon against COVID-19: Trust." *BMJ*, no. 371 (Dec. 11, 2020). https://www.bmj.com/content/371/bmj.m4720.

Cameron, Elizabeth E., Jennifer B. Nuzzo, and Jessica A. Bell. *Global Health Security Index: Building Collective Action and Accountability*, report. Washington, DC: Nuclear Threat Initiative, October 2019. https://www.ghsindex.org/wp-content/uploads/2020/04/2019-Global-Health-Security-Index.pdf.

Carter, David P., and Peter J. May. "Making Sense of the U.S. COVID-19 Pandemic Response: A Policy Regime Perspective." *Administrative Theory and Praxis* 42, no. 2 (2020): 265–77.

Clifford, James. "Spatial Practices: Fieldwork, Travel, and the Disciplining of Anthropology." In *Anthropological Locations: Boundaries and Grounds of a Field Science*, edited by Akhil Gupta and James Ferguson, 185–222. Berkeley: University of California Press, 1997.

Cohen, Matthew. "The Rise in Testing Is Not Driving the Rise in U.S. Virus Cases." *New York Times*, July 22, 2020. https://www.nytimes.com/interactive/2020/07/22/us/covid-testing-rising-cases.html.

"The COVD-19 Infodemic." *Lancet Infectious Diseases* 20, no. 8 (Aug. 2020): 875.

Cullen, Art. *Storm Lake: A Chronicle of Change, Resilience, and Hope from a Heartland Newspaper*. New York: Penguin, 2018.

Cummings, Christine. "After Glitch Fix, Experts Still Have Questions about State Coronavirus Data." *Iowa News Now*, Aug. 26, 2020. https://cbs2iowa.com/news/local/after-glitch-fix-experts-still-have-questions-about-state-coronavirus-data.

Djupe, Paul A., and Ryan P. Burge. "Trump the Anointed?" *Religion in Public: Exploring the Mix of Sacred and Secular* (blog), May 11, 2020. https://religioninpublic.blog/2020/05/11/trump-the-anointed.

Diamond, Dan, Tyler Pager, and Jeff Stein. "Biden Commits to Waiving Vaccine Patents, Driving Wedge with Pharmaceutical Companies." *Washington Post*, May 5, 2021. https://www.washingtonpost.com/health/2021/05/05/biden-waives-vaccine-patents.

Dias, Elizabeth, and Ruth Graham. "White Evangelical Resistance Is Obstacle in Vaccine Effort." *New York Times*, April 12, 2021. https://www.nytimes.com/2021/04/05/us/covid-vaccine-evangelicals.html.

Duffy, Molly. "Gov. Kim Reynolds Orders Iowa Schools to 'Take All Efforts' to Get Kids Back in Classrooms." *Gazette* (Iowa), July 17, 2020. https://www.thegazette.com/subject/news/education/gov-kim-reynolds-to-direct-all-iowa-schools-to-reopen-in-person-when-school-year-begins-next-month-20200717.

Dyer, Owen. "Covid-19: Many Poor Countries Will See Almost No Vaccine Next Year, Aid Groups Warn." *BMJ*, no. 371 (Dec. 11, 2021): m2809. https://www.bmj.com/content/371/bmj.m4809.

Dzhurova, Albena. "Symbolic Politics and Government Response to a National Emergency: Narrating the COVID-19 Crisis." *Administrative Theory and Praxis* 42, no. 4 (2020): 571–87. DOI: 10.1080/10841806.2020.1816787.

Eaton, Lisa A., and Seth C. Kalichman. "Social and Behavioral Health Responses to COVID-19: Lessons Learned from Four Decades of the HIV Pandemic." *Journal of Behavioral Medicine* 43, no. 3 (June 2020): 341–45. DOI: 10.1007/s10865-020-00157-y.

Edwards, Johnny. "Some Chiropractors Stoke Fear of Covid Vaccine." *Seattle Times*, May 24, 2021. https://www.seattletimes.com/seattle-news/health/some-chiropractors-stoking-fear-of-covid-vaccines.

Eggertson, Laura. "Lancet Retracts 12-Year-Old Article Linking Autism to MMR Vaccines." *Canadian Medical Association Journal* 182, no. 4 (2010): E199–E200.

Elston, Hattie P. *White Men Follow After: A Collection of Stories about the Okoboji-Spirit Lake Region.* Spirit Lake, IA: Dickinson County Historical Society and Museum, 1988.

Epstein, Steve. *Impure Science: AIDS, Activism, and the Politics of Knowledge.* Berkeley: University of California Press, 1998.

Erikson, Erik H. *Childhood and Society,* 2nd ed. New York: Norton, 1993.

Farmer, Paul. *AIDS and Accusation: Haiti and the Geography of Blame.* Berkeley: University of California Press, 1992.

Farmer, Paul, Arthur Kleinman, Jim Y. Kim., and Matthew Basilico. *Reimagining Global Health: An Introduction.* Berkeley: University of California Press, 2013.

Fischer, Julie, and Rebecca Katz. "U.S. Priorities for Global Health Security." In *Global Health Policy in the Second Obama Term: A Report of the CSIS Global Health Policy Center,* edited by J. Stephen Morrison, 85–95. Washington, DC: Global Health Policy Center, 2013.

Foley, Ryan. "'Horrifying' Data Glitch Skews Key Iowa Coronavirus Metrics." *Gazette* (Iowa), Aug. 17, 2020. https://www.thegazette.com/subject/news/government/iowa-covid-data-glitch-metrics-schools-percent-positive-20200817.

Foley, Ryan. "Iowa Governor's Push to Reopen Schools Descends into Chaos." *AP News,* Aug. 19, 2020. https://apnews.com/article/319e899fe751d462fe3576c4010fb642.

Fraser, Caroline. *Prairie Fires: The American Dreams of Laura Ingles Wilder.* New York: Metropolitan Books, 2017.

Fukuyama, Francis. *Identity: The Demand for Dignity and the Politics of Resentment.* New York: Farrar, Strauss, Giroux, 2018.

Funk, Cary, and Alec Tyson. "Growing Share of Americans Say They Plan to Get a COVID-19 Vaccine—or Already Have." Pew Research Center, March 5, 2021. https://www.pewresearch.org/science/2021/03/05/growing-share-of-americans-say-they-plan-to-get-a-covid-19-vaccine-or-already-have.

Gardner-Sharp, Abbie. *History of the Spirit Lake Massacre and Captivity of Miss Abbie Gardner.* Des Moines, IA: Wallace-Homestead Book, 1885.

Ghebreyesus, Tedros Adhanom. "Acting on NCDs: Counting the Cost." *Lancet* 391, no. 10134 (May 19, 2018): 1973–73. https://doi.org/10.1016/S0140-6736(18)30675-5.

Godfrey, Elaine. "Iowa Is What Happens When Government Does Nothing." *The Atlantic*, Dec. 3, 2020. https://www.theatlantic.com/politics/archive/2020/12/how-iowa-mishandled-coronavirus-pandemic/617252.

Gostin, Lawrence, and Rebecca Katz. "The International Health Regulations: The Governing Framework for Global Health Security." *Milbank Quarterly* 94, no. 2 (2016): 264–313.

Grant, Adam. "There's a Name for the Blah You're Feeling: It's Called Languishing." *New York Times*, April 19, 2021. https://www.nytimes.com/2021/04/19/well/mind/covid-mental-health-languishing.html.

Greenwood, Lee. "God Bless the U.S.A." *You've Got a Good Love Comin'*. MCA Records, 1984.

Grieder, Jonathan, Ross Grooters, Pat Morrissey, Mazahir Salih, Chris Schwartz, and Stacey Walker. "COVID-19 Response Should Protect Working Communities. Why Is the Governor Putting Corporate Profits First?" *Des Moines Register*, July 6, 2020. https://www.desmoinesregister.com/story/opinion/columnists/iowa-view/2020/07/06/local-iowa-officials-reynolds-has-wrong-priorities-covid-19-response/5360779002.

Haidt, Jonathan. *The Righteous Mind: Why Good People are Divided by Politics and Religion*. New York: Vintage, 2012.

Hardy, Bradley L., and Trevon D. Logan. *Racial Economic Inequality amid the COVID-19 Crisis*. The Hamilton Project, Essay 2020-17. Washington, DC: Brookings, August 2020. https://www.brookings.edu/wp-content/uploads/2020/08/EA_Hardy-Logan_LO_8.12.pdf.

Hoganson, Kristin L. *The Heartland: An American History*. New York: Penguin Press, 2019.

Hytek, Nick. "COVID-19 Trends Rise across State, but not in Northwest Iowa." *Sioux City Journal*, July 25, 2020. https://siouxcityjournal.com/news/local/covid-19-trends-rise-across-

state-but-not-in-northwest-iowa/article_f15b5058–87db-
5b8b-8531-ec14c8d98fcc.html.

Kashen, Julie, Sarah Jane Glynn, and Amanda Novello. "How
COVID-19 Sent Women's Workforce Progress Backward." Center
for American Progress, October 30, 2020. https://www.
americanprogress.org/issues/women/reports/2020/10/30/
492582/covid-19-sent-womens-workforce-progress-backward.

Keith-Jennings, Brynne. "Food Need Very High Compared to
Pre-Pandemic Levels, Making Relief Imperative." *Off the Charts*
(blog), Center on Budget and Policy Priorities, Sept. 10, 2020.
https://www.cbpp.org/blog/food-need-very-high-compared-to-
pre-pandemic-levels-making-relief-imperative.

Kenworthy, Nora, Adam Koon, and Emily Mendenhall. "On Symbols
and Scripts: The Politics of the American COVID-19 Response."
Global Public Health 16, no. 8-9 (March 19, 2021): 1424–38. DOI:
10.1080/17441692.2021.1902549.

Khazan, Olga. "How a Bizarre Claim about Masks Has Lived on for
Months." *The Atlantic*, Oct. 9, 2020. https://www.
theatlantic.com/politics/archive/2020/10/can-masks-make-you-
sicker/616641.

Konyndyk, Jeremy. "Global Health Security in the Trump Era: Time
to Worry?" *Commentary and Analysis* (blog), Center for Global
Development, May 17, 2018. https://www.cgdev.org/blog/global-
health-security-trump-era-time-worry.

Lamott, Anne. *Bird by Bird: Some Instructions on Writing and Life.*
New York: Anchor Books, 1994.

Lanoo, Michael J. *The Iowa Lakeside Laboratory: A Century of Discovering the Nature of Nature.* Iowa City: University of Iowa Press, 2012.

Larson, Heidi. *Stuck: How Vaccine Rumors Start—and Why They
Don't Go Away.* Oxford, UK: Oxford University Press, 2020.

Ledford, Heidi. "Moderna COVID Vaccine Becomes Second to Get
US Authorization: Two RNA Vaccines Will Be Useful as US
Infections Surge, but the Speedy Authorizations Complicate
Clinical Trials." *Nature*, Dec. 18, 2020. https://www.nature.com/
articles/d41586-020-03593-7.

Lemonick, Michael D., and Alice Park. "The Truth about SARS." *Time*, May 5, 2003. http://content.time.com/time/subscriber/article/0,33009,1004763,00.html.

Levitz, Eric. "Trump Condemns New York for Planning Ahead on Coronavirus." *New York Magazine: Intelligencer*, March 30, 2020. https://nymag.com/intelligencer/2020/03/coronavirus-trump-new-york-ventilators-cuomo.html.

Lévi-Strauss, Claude. *The Savage Mind*. Chicago: University of Chicago Press, 1966. First published as *La Pensée sauvage*, Paris: Librairie Plon, 1962.

Leys, Tony. "Gov. Kim Reynolds Says Iowans Can Trust State's Coronavirus Data, Despite History of Glitches." *Des Moines Register*, Sept. 2, 2020. https://www.desmoinesregister.com/story/news/health/2020/09/02/governor-kim-reynolds-iowa-covid-19-data-trustworthy-despite-glitches/5695310002.

Leys, Tony, and Stephen Gruber-Miller. "Kim Reynolds Defends Iowa's COVID Data Credibility, Claims Transparency after 'Glitch' Skewed Official Numbers." *Des Moines Register*, Aug. 20, 2020. https://www.desmoinesregister.com/story/news/health/2020/08/20/iowa-health-leaders-fix-backdating-glitch-coronavirus-data-reports/5612558002.

Litt, Eden, and Eszter Hargittai. "The Imagined Audience on Social Network Sites." *Social Medica + Society* 2, no. 1 (January–March 2016): 1–12.

Manderson, Lenore, and Susan Levine. "COVID-19, Risk, Fear, and Fall-Out." *Medical Anthropology* 39, no. 5 (2020): 367–70.

Mendenhall, Emily. "How an Iowa Summer Resort Region Became a COVID-19 Hot Spot." *Vox*, August 8, 2020. https://www.vox.com/2020/8/8/21357625/covid-19-iowa-lakes-okoboji-kim-reynolds-masks.

Mendenhall, Emily. *Rethinking Diabetes: Entanglements with Trauma, Poverty, and HIV*. Ithaca, NY: Cornell University Press, 2019.

Mendenhall, Emily. *Syndemic Suffering: Social Distress, Depression, and Diabetes among Mexican Immigrant Women*. New York: Routledge, 2012.

Metzl, Jonathan. *Dying of Whiteness: How the Politics of Racial Resentment Is Killing America's Heartland*. New York: Basic Books, 2019.

Michel, Lawrence, Josh Bivens, Elise Gould, and Heidi Shierholz. *The State of Working America*, 12th ed. Ithaca, NY: Economic Policy Institute book published by Cornell University Press, 2012. http://www.stateofworkingamerica.org/subjects/income/index.html.

Mitchell, Russ. "Iowa Supreme Court Issues 'Fish House Lounge' Ruling." *Dickinson County News*, April 26, 2013. https://siouxcityjournal.com/business/okoboji-businessman-files-lawsuit-against-city-council/article_86036b56-d53f-5ca4-a40c-ff7e167509c7.html.

Mol, Annemarie. *The Logic of Care: Health and the Problem of Patient Choice*. New York: Routledge, 2008.

Molteni, Mega. "Iowa's Covid Wave and the Limits of Personal Responsibility." *Wired*, November 20, 2020. https://www.wired.com/story/iowas-covid-wave-and-the-limits-of-personal-responsibility.

Moreland, Amanda, et al., "Timing of State and Territorial COVID-19 Stay-at-Home Orders and Changes in Population Movement—United States, March 1–May 31, 2020." *Morbidity and Mortality Weekly Report* 69, no. 35 (September 4, 2020): 1198–203. https://www.cdc.gov/mmwr/volumes/69/wr/mm6935a2.htm.

Nephew, Lauren D. "Systemic Racism and Overcoming My COVID-19 Vaccine Hesitancy." *EClinicalMedicine* 32 (Feb. 1, 2021): 100713. https://doi.org/10.1016/j.eclinm.2020.100713.

Nicholas, Peter, and Kathy Gilsinan. "The End of the Imperial Presidency." *The Atlantic*, May 2, 2020. https://www.theatlantic.com/politics/archive/2020/05/trump-governors-coronavirus/611023.

Nicholas, Peter, and Ed Yong. "Fauci: 'Bizarre' White House Behavior Only Hurts the President." *The Atlantic*, July 15, 2020. https://www.theatlantic.com/politics/archive/2020/07/trump-fauci-coronavirus-pandemic-oppo/614224.

Nyabola, Nanjala. "How to Talk about COVID-19 in Africa." *Boston Review*, Oct. 15, 2020. http://bostonreview.net/ global-justice/nanjala-nyabola-how-talk-about-covid-19-africa.

Oak Lake Writers Society, Craig Howe, and Kim TallBear, eds. *This Stretch of River*. Sioux Falls, SD: Pine Hill Press, 2006.

Packard, Randall. *A History of Global Health: Interventions into the Lives of Other Peoples*. Baltimore, MD: Johns Hopkins University Press, 2016.

Papacharissi, Zizi. *Affective Publics: Sentiment, Technology, and Politics*. Oxford, UK: Oxford University Press, 2014.

Parsons, John. *Inkpaduta and the Sioux Indians*. Spirit Lake, IA: Okoboji Protective Association, 1998.

Paz, Christian. "All the President's Lies about the Coronavirus: An Unfinished Compendium of Trump's Overwhelming Dishonesty during a National Emergency. *The Atlantic*, Nov. 2, 2020. https://www.theatlantic.com/politics/archive/2020/11/trumps-lies-about-coronavirus/608647.

Pfannenstiel, Brianne, and Nick Coltrain. "Gov. Kim Reynolds Says Iowa Will Loosen Restrictions on the Economy This Week." *Des Moines Register*, May 11, 2020. https://www.desmoinesregister.com/story/news/health/2020/05/11/iowa-gov-kim-reynolds-covid-19-coronavirus-data-matrix-maps-reopening/3073063001.

Pfannenstiel, Brianne, and Nick Coltrain. "Iowa Gov. Kim Reynolds Taking Extra Precautions, State Epidemiologist Quarantining after Potential Coronavirus Exposure at White House." *Des Moines Register*, May 11, 2020. https://www.desmoinesregister.com/story/news/politics/2020/05/11/iowa-gov-reynolds-extra-precautions-white-house-visit-coronavirus-exposure-mike-pence/3106601001

Phelan, Alexandra L., and Lawrence Gostin. "Law as a Fixture between the One Health Interfaces of Emerging Diseases." *Transactions of the Royal Society of Tropical Medicine and Hygiene* 111, no. 6 (2017): 241–43. doi: 10.1093/trstmh/trx044.

Phelan, Alexandra L., Rebecca Katz, and Lawrence O. Gostin. "The Novel Coronavirus Originating in Wuhan, China." *JAMA* 323, no. 8 (Jan. 30, 2020): 709–10. https://jamanetwork.com/journals/jama/fullarticle/2760500.

Prout, Katie. "A History of Violence: Walking the Blood-Soaked Shores of Spirit Lake: Rethinking an Early-American Captivity

Narrative." *Lit Hub*, March 1, 2017. https://lithub.com/crime-or-conflict-walking-the-blood-soaked-shores-of-spirit-lake.

Qiaoan, Runya. "The Myth of Masks: A Tale of Risk Selection in the COVID-19 Pandemic." "Forum on COVID-19 Pandemic," special issue of *Social Anthropology* 28, no. 2 (May 2020): 336–37. https://onlinelibrary.wiley.com/doi/10.1111/1469-8676.12852.

Ramey, Larry, and Daniel Haley. *Tackling Giants: The Life Story of Berkley Bedell*. Loveland, CO: National Foundation of Alternative Medicine, 2005.

Reich, Adam, and Peter Bearman. *Working for Respect: Community and Conflict at Walmart*. Ithaca, NY: Columbia University Press, 2018.

Reich, Jennifer. "Neoliberal Mothering and Vaccine Refusal: Imagined Gated Communities and the Privilege of Choice." *Gender and Society* 28, no. 5 (2014): 679–704.

Reich, Jennifer. "'We Are Fierce, Independent Thinkers and Intelligent': Social Capital and Stigma Management among Mothers Who Refuse Vaccines." *Social Science and Medicine* 257 (July 2020): 112015.

Roose, Kevin. "What Is QAnon, the Viral Pro-Trump Conspiracy Theory?" *New York Times*, Feb. 4, 2021. https://www.nytimes.com/article/what-is-qanon.html.

Ryan, Michael. "Dr. Alfred Katz Says Fear, Not Aids, Is Causing a Red Cross Blood Loss." *People Magazine*, July 11, 1983. https://people.com/archive/dr-alfred-katz-says-fear-not-aids-is-causing-a-red-cross-blood-loss-vol-20-no-2.

Sangaramoorthy, Thurka, and Adia Benton. "Imagining Rural Immunity." *Anthropology News*, June 19, 2020. https://www.anthropology-news.org/index.php/2020/06/19/imagining-rural-immunity.

Schilts, Randy. *And the Band Played On: Politics, People, and the AIDS Epidemic*. New York: St Martin's Griffin, 1987.

Senior, Jennifer. "I Spoke with Anthony Fauci. He Says His Inbox Isn't Pretty." *New York Times*, July 21, 2020. https://www.nytimes.com/2020/07/21/opinion/anthony-fauci-coronavirus.html.

"'The Skunk at the Picnic': Dr. Anthony Fauci on Working for Trump."
The Daily, *New York Times*, Jan. 26, 2020. https://www.
nytimes.com/2021/01/26/podcasts/the-daily/anthony-fauci-
donald-trump-coronavirus-pandemic.html.

Smarsh, Sarah. *Heartland: A Memoir of Working Hard and Being
Broke in the Richest Country on Earth*. New York: Scribner, 2019.

Smith, Christen A. "Facing the Dragon: Black Mothering, Sequelae,
and Gendered Necropolitics in the Americas." *Transforming
Anthropology* 24, no. 1 (2016): 31–48.

Smith, Philip, Susan Chu, and Lawrence Barker. "Children Who
Have Received No Vaccines: Who Are They and Where Do They
Live?" *Pediatrics* 114, no. 1 (July 2004): 187–95. DOI: https://doi.
org/10.1542/peds.114.1.187.

Sobo, Elisa J. "Social Cultivation of Vaccine Refusal and Delay
among Waldorf (Steiner) School Parents." *Medical Anthropology
Quarterly* 29 no. 3 (2015): 381–99.

Sobo, Elisa J. "Theorizing (Vaccine) Refusal: Through the Looking
Glass." *Cultural Anthropology* 31, no. 3 (2016): 342–50.

Sobo, EJ (Elisa J). "Playing with Conspiracy Theories." *Anthropology
News*, July 31, 2020. https://doi.org/10.1111/AN.1236.

Soutard, Dargan. "Tyson Meat Plant in Storm Lake to Shut Down
Temporarily after State Confirms Coronavirus Outbreak." *Des
Moines Register*, May 28, 2020. https://www.desmoinesregister.
com/story/news/politics/2020/05/28/coronavirus-outbreak-
confirmed-tyson-foods-storm-lake-pork-processing-plant-
kim-reynolds/5274618002.

Sparke, Matthew, and Dimitar Anguelov. "Contextualising Coronavirus Geographically." *Transactions of the Institute of British
Geographers* 45, no. 3 (Sept. 2020): 498–508.

Ta, Lindh. "Reynolds Shifts Tone, Requires Masks Indoor as Hospitalizations Skyrocket." *Iowa Capital Dispatch*, Nov. 16, 2020. https://
iowacapitaldispatch.com/2020/11/16/reynolds-shifts-tone-
requires-masks-indoor-as-hospitalizations-skyrocket.

Temkar, Arvin. "My Fellow Liberals Hate Lee Greenwood's 'God
Bless the USA.'; I Love It." *Washington Post*, June 30, 2017.

https://www.washingtonpost.com/outlook/my-fellow-liberals-hate-lee-greenwoods-god-bless-the-usa-i-love-it/2017/06/30/e09ce46a-5a9f-11e7–9fc6-c7ef4bc58d13_story.html.

Ungar, Laura. "More Women Than Men Are Getting COVID Vaccines." *Scientific American*, April 12, 2021. https://www.scientificamerican.com/article/more-women-than-men-are-getting-covid-vaccines.

Wakefield, A., S. H. Murch, A. Anthony, J. Linnell, D. M. Casson, M. Malik, M. Berelowitz, A. P. Dillon, M. A. Thomson, P. Harvey, A. Valentine, S. E. Davies, J. A. Walker-Smith. "RETRACTED: Ileal-Lymphoid-Nodular Hyperplasia, Non-Specific Colitis, and Pervasive Developmental Disorder in Children." *Lancet* 351, no. 9103 (1998): 637–41.

Westerman, Gwen, and Bruce White. *Mni Sota Makoce: The Land of the Dakota*. St Paul: Minnesota Historical Society Press, 2012.

Wills, John. "When Should Iowa Reopen the Economy?" *Dickinson County News*, April 28, 2020. https://www.dickinsoncountynews.com/story/2686550.html.

Wills, John. "It's Time to Return Lost Rights." *Dickinson County News*, May 19, 2020. https://www.dickinsoncountynews.com/story/2810675.html.

Wilson, Suze. "Three Reasons Why Jacinda Ardern's Coronavirus Response Has Been a Masterclass in Crisis Leadership." *The Conversation*, April 5, 2020. http://theconversation.com/three-reasons-why-jacinda-arderns-coronavirus-response-has-been-a-masterclass-in-crisis-leadership-135541.

Woulter, Doug. "Sibley-Ocheyedan Football Team Battles Coronavirus, Hopes to Forge Winning Tradition." *Globe* (Worthington, MN), Sept. 30, 2020. https://www.dglobe.com/sports/6681654-Sibley-Ocheyedan-football-team-battles-coronavirus-hopes-to-forge-winning-tradition.

Yasmin, Seema. *Viral BS: Medical Myths and Why We Fall for Them*. Baltimore, MD: Johns Hopkins University Press, 2021.

Zauzmer, Julie. "Following the Pittsburgh Attack, Rep. Steve King's Iowa Supporters Brush Aside Concern about His White Nation-

alist Views." *The Washington Post*, October 28, 2018. https://
www.washingtonpost.com/politics/in-the-wake-of-the-
pittsburgh-attack-rep-steve-kings-iowa-supporters-brush-aside-
concern-about-his-white-nationalist-views/2018/10/28/
a16b7044-dabf-11e8-b732–3c72cbf131f2_story.html.

INDEX

Page numbers in *italics* refer to illustrations.

Index